COVID AND VACCINES FOR THE COMMON MAN

Covid and Vaccines For The Common Man

Kelly Gregg MD

TABLE OF CONTENTS

INTRODUCTION

I started writing about Diet and Health a few years ago. It started with the observation that there were lots of people with type 2 diabetes. . It turns out that this is related to obesity. In fact, over 40% of the adults in the US had obesity, prediabetes, or type 2 diabetes. That seemed to be a high number.

When I examined history, it was not always like this. Whatever was causing this seemed to have appeared in the last couple hundred years. Eventually, I determined it was not a lack of exercise or an excess of food in the world, it was the diet.

The modern western diet has induced obesity in every modern country who has adopted this diet. This led me to write numerous books and my having to teach people about diabetes, eating, fasting, metabolism, and of course diet. I then realized I had to start in the womb, which has led to books about epigenetics in pregnancy.

The point is that this started with an accepted observation, but I wanted to know why this was the case.

Now I have the chart below, that is deaths from covid since Jan 2020. I am living through this history. I remember when there was not a vaccine. Early in 2020 there was a peak of infections in New York City in which the hospitals were jammed. People were dying in the hallways and emergency rooms. There was no treatment except supportive care and ventilators, and that did not work well at all. Basically no one knew what was happening or what was going to happen.

We reverted to the historical treatment for epidemics which was to quarantine the sick. For some reason we thought masking everyone would protect us, despite our only masking sick people in previous epidemics. Of course, it was soon evident that the old and immune compromised were at a much-increased risk, the same as it had been in all epidemics. Even though we also soon discovered children did not appear to be at high risk, we closed the schools. This was something we had also done in past epidemics.

We had no vaccine, no medications, no real treatment, and a severe respiratory virus that we had not seen before. It was starting to sound like the Spanish Flu of 1918 all over again. The only way we got over that one was to wait for herd immunity at the cost of numerous lives.

You remember we shut down businesses for two weeks to flatten the curve. Now we wonder if that worked or was even a good idea, but I agreed at the time with that approach. Now I do not think that was a good idea, but hindsight is 20/20.

People were wearing masks, segregating, and staying at home; Some voluntary, some mandated. Various treatments were being tried with slight success. We were waiting for a new vaccine which was supposed to offer some hope.

The vaccine was approved in Dec 2020. This was right around the peak in the daily number of covid deaths in the US. See chart. People were standing in line to get one. We were smart enough to prioritize the elderly as they were obviously at increased risk. Another vaccine was approved in Jan 2021. The supply chain was functioning and now the CDC is on TV telling us to get the vaccine in order to stop the spread of covid and thus get us to develop herd immunity. Of course, most people were already trying to get a vaccine.

Just as we all should have been rejoicing that we had a handle on the epidemic and life would return to normal, it takes a bad turn.

The government, both state and federal, begins demanding you must get the vaccine, something we had not done before. Why would we have to do that? You would have to be crazy not to get the vaccine, or maybe not.

Every adult in the US knew what a vaccine was from personal experience. We got tetanus vaccines, we got MMR, if you were old enough you had gotten a smallpox vaccine. Many had gotten flu vaccines. We thought if you got a vaccine, it protected you from getting the disease. Sure, we knew it wasn't perfect, but what is.

Now we had a new type of vaccine, and it was not crazy to expect it would work like any other vaccine. The CDC was telling us this every day. I and many other physicians were a little concerned in that we knew that a normal vaccine takes years to get approved. We knew that it would take a million people getting the vaccine and watching them for a year to be sure it was safe. And this was no normal vaccine. We really had no experience with it.

But this was an emergency and it got emergency authorization for temporary approval. We knew there was a slight risk, but for the most part for most people, the risk was probably worth the benefit. Nobody really complained too much.

Then it became mandated. That bothered some people. By now I know that if I am in good health, my risk of dying from covid is low. At the same time, I don't want to get sick or have to go to the hospital, so it is probably worth it. But to make me get the vaccine whether I want it or not, well, that just doesn't sound right.

The CDC on TV every day told me I had to get it otherwise grandma could catch it from you and die. I don't want grandma to die, but she got the vaccine two months ago. Why then do I have to get the vaccine to keep her from dying?

Suddenly I am starting to wonder is this new vaccine is really a vaccine. It started to sound a lot more like the gamma globulin shot we used to give years ago. It would keep you from getting sick for a while, and help you if you were sick, but it was no vaccine.

Now it's July 10, 2021. The new vaccine has been out about six months. I am looking at the graph the CDC puts out every week and I see cases and deaths from covid are at the lowest level they have been at for over a year. The vaccine appears to be working. I may not like it, but I can't argue with success. I may not like being forced to get the shot, but I plan to go along.

Today is a year later. I am looking at the chart. I don't understand what is going on. I still can remember how everyone getting forced to get the vaccine was going to be worth it. Is the current graph what all the experts predicted?

I'm back to the time when I was wondering why everyone is getting fat and getting diabetes. I eventually figured that out and what to do about it. Many other people were doing the same thing and there are thousands of diet books. Where are all the people explaining to me why the chart looks like this and what to do about it? Can you tell me what the chart is going to look like six months from now?

When I think back over the last year or so, I remembered that I did not read much about people questioning the effectiveness of the vaccine. Certainly not any debate. I know now there actually were people, it's just those opinions were being suppressed.; by the print media, the social media, the television media, and the state and federal governments. Physicians were being disciplined for spreading false information. Websites were shut down, People were taken off Facebook, contrary opinions were either not published anywhere or ridiculed, maybe denounced as unpatriotic. I know there were physicians that did not agree with mandating vaccines, but you could not find them.

Without a vaccine or antiviral medications, it took about two years to get herd immunity for the Spanish Flue 1918-1920. We are now at almost three years with covid and no sign of herd immunity.

Dr. Bossche has written a paper trying to answer the question as to why the new vaccines have not solved the covid problem. The paper is difficult to read and therefore few are going to read it.

It appears that the paper was written to a somewhat select group of people, that is, those involved in covid and vaccine research. He has put forth a theory and he is trying to convince these people it is true. In this 45-page paper he has included over 120 citations. The argument assumes prior knowledge of the language of virology and vaccines. It is also sometimes difficult to follow . The common man simply does not know the language.

I have read the paper numerous times. It takes me awhile to get through it as I must look up many things I don't understand, never learned, forgot about, or to get a definition. I am not an expert in this field, but I will probably be the only one to actually look up all the references. I say look up but on my pdf copy on my computer, I just click on the reference.

I am not an expert, but despite the media dismissing his ideas, everyone who looks at his resume would consider Dr Bossche to be one. He is not an academic and does not work in an ivory tower. He has worked at real jobs.

Although I am a retired physician and have not personally examined him, he is not a wacko. He does not do a decent job presenting his ideas to the common man. That is not surprising as this paper is not written for laymen. In all my books I believe the common man using common sense can understand most of these concepts if I just teach him the language of the subject. That is my job and that is what I am going to do with this book for this paper.

I want to answer the question; why does the covid cases, hospitalizations, and death charts look like they do? What does that mean, and what can we expect?

I do not reproduce the paper and have given you the link to look it up yourself. If you want to get the references, you will have to get the paper. I have written another book in which I reproduce his paper and go through it line by line. I look up every reference. I often must add my own explanatory comments and add paragraphs of my own explanatory notes. . I may have clarified it for a few more people who had a solid understanding of the subject. I am talking about graduates in biological science. I think I may have succeeded in explaining it to most physicians.

My job has always been to explain things to the common man. I will accomplish this by giving some necessary background and summarizing the conclusions. This will still take a while. I will give you Dr. Bossche's conclusions. At the end of the book, I will give my conclusions.

It is now eleven months since I first published this book. Nothing in my conclusions have changed. The incidence is low, but covid is still circulating around the world and no one would say herd immunity is present. As expected, several variants have arisen. Also as expected, the vaccine does not keep you from getting covid.

Even those at the CDC must now admit that the vaccine, nor the boosters, are effective in preventing covid. Now they emphasize that the reason to get the vaccine is to prevent dying from covid. I still stand by my explanation why this is so. Actually, this is Dr. Bossche's explanation, but I still support it.

The CDC still advises everyone to get the vaccine but lacks any explanation how getting the vaccine will prevent severe disease. They do not seem to address the issue how a vaccine can prevent dying but cannot prevent you from getting the disease; something unheard of in previous vaccines.

Although covid persists, there still has not been a variant arise which has an increased mortality. In other words, one which avoids the antibody which prevents systemic spread. I am not hoping it does arise, after all both me and almost everyone I know has been vaccinated. I still believe the vaccinated will be at a disadvantage as far as survival compared to the unvaccinated who caught the virus.

Over the last year we have verified aspects of the vaccine which I only thought may be true. We also have learned much about Long Covid, and now believe this is related to the mRNA vaccine more so than the covid virus. Misinformation, the wrong information, lies about the mRNA vaccine, and suppression of any dissent is now clear. The CDC and FDA knows this but still will only vaguely indicate that they were quite wrong in approving this for emergency use and that the vaccine itself has caused harm to many.

Previously I only indicated that the covid virus was likely from the Wuhan lab and that it was genetically manipulated to be both more infective and have an increased mutation rate. Now most believe this is the case. Yet academics continue to treat this as a natural virus and base predictions on this rather that realizing the manipulated virus is not acting like a normal virus.

I still stand by my previous prediction and previous recommendations, but I hope I am wrong.

KELLY GREGG MD

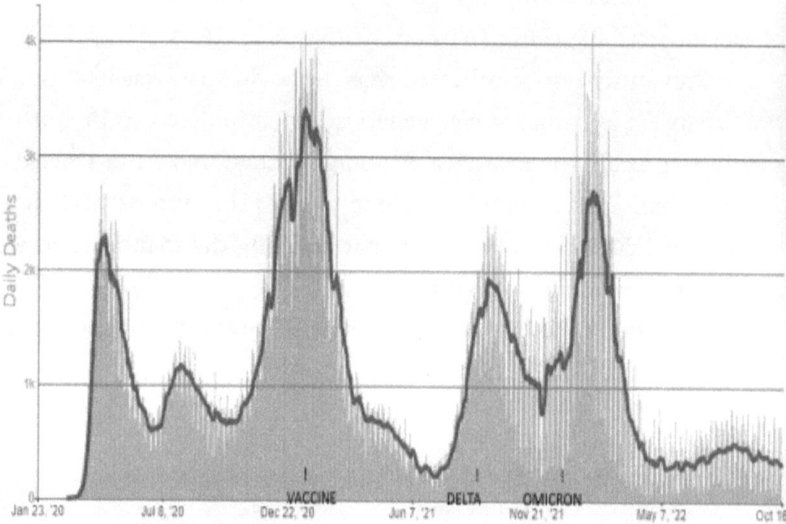

Daily Trends in Number of COVID-19 Deaths in The United States Reported to CDC

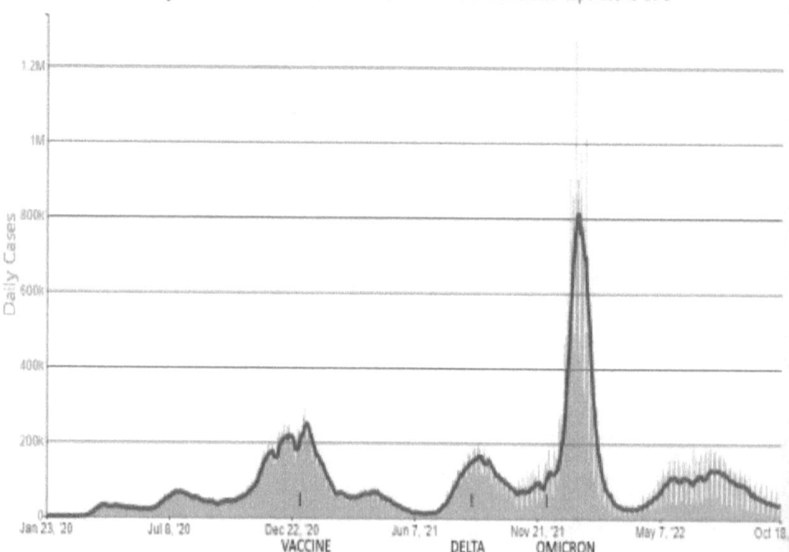

Daily Trends in Number of COVID-19 Cases in The United States Reported to CDC

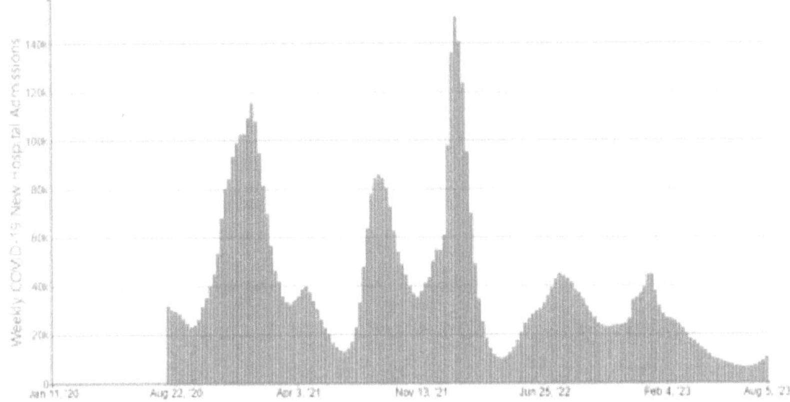

Centers for Disease Control and Prevention. COVID Data Tracker. Atlanta, GA: U.S. Department of Health and Human Services, CDC; 2023, August 16. https://covid.cdc.gov/covid-data-tracker

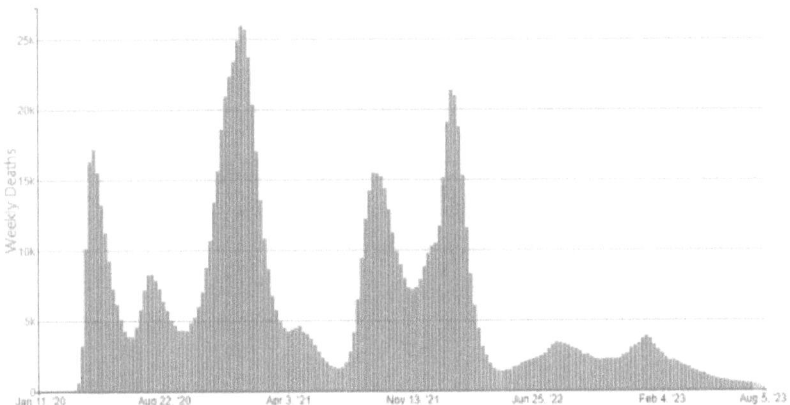

Centers for Disease Control and Prevention. COVID Data Tracker. Atlanta, GA: U.S. Department of Health and Human Services, CDC; 2023, August 16. https://covid.cdc.gov/covid-data-tracker

Above you can see an updated deaths graph. The CDC has changed the presentation of the graphs somewhat, but the death data is the same. Deaths are a solid statistic since every death is accompanied by paperwork and is searchable.

It has become almost useless to calculate the incidence of covid since the disease has become so mild that most do not even get a test, and those who do get a test do not report the results to anyone.

It is much more useful to follow hospital admissions as these patient have gotten symptomatic covid with a positive test and the results are reported. Hence this become a better metric to see if the incidence is increasing.

Of course the incidence and the number of deaths should mirror each other, but we can still see if the mortality is increasing dramatically.

Unless the mortality increases, there is no cause for urgent alarm. But the charts also show herd immunity has still not occurred after 3 ½ years as we expect it should have if the were a normal pandemic and a normal virus. Covid is still circulating in the population and still mutating.

<u>Review</u>

I have written numerous books on Diet and Health. All of these are nonfiction, which means they are based upon my study of the subjects through books written by many others who may have a much greater expertise in these matters. Usually, I have come to conclusions based upon my lifetime accumulation of knowledge and experiences, as well as looking at the same material as others but explaining it differently.

This is the way almost all nonfiction books are created. I have not discovered new information but interpreted it in a different manner. In addition, I have developed a method of teaching this information so as the common man can understand it.

Again, nothing new. Every math teacher starts out with the same information, yet some are much better at teaching math than others.

I wrote a lunchtime Kindle book on artificial sweeteners based on a paper:

Artificial sweeteners induce glucose intolerance by altering the gut microbiota Jotham Suez, Tal Korem, et al., Nature 514, 181-188 (2014)

I certainly did not claim that I did any of this work nor arrived at conclusions, but rather tried to explain the data and how this related to Diet and Health. Similarly, this book is going to be an explanation of a paper which is much longer and more difficult to understand. That paper is:

Poor virus-neutralizing capacity in highly C-19 vaccinated populations could soon lead to a fulminate spread of SARs-CoV-2 super variants that are highly infections and highly virulent in vaccinees while being fully resistant to all existing and future spike-based C-19 vaccines. Geert Vanden Bossche DVD, PhD, voiceforscienceandsolidarity.org

https://uploads-ssl.webflow.com/616004c52e87ed08692f5692/627933433cc6dc1c869df8ad_GVB%27s%20analysis%20of%20C-19%20c

Like the rest of the world, I knew very little about Covid 2.5 years ago. That is not to say I was ignorant about viruses or epidemics, in fact I may have known slightly more than most physicians and almost all laymen as I have time to read more, but I was nowhere close to having any extensive knowledge. I was able for the most part to speak the language in that area and half-way understand what people were talking about.

At the same time, 2.5 years ago I had high regard for the CDC and FDA and had a pretty good knowledge of the logistics of clinical trials. Like almost all physicians I trusted the CDC.

Most of us remember the time frame. There was a new infective virus of which not much was known. There was no vaccine, and no effective chemical prophylaxis or treatment. For many years we had been used to periodic influenza epidemics and usually people did not have unusual fear. Usually, we treated these similar to the way people had done for years. If you are sick, stay home. If you think someone is sick, stay away from them. Practice good general hygiene and handwashing. For the past fifty years or so some sort of vaccine was available. Taking the vaccine was advised. Now we know it is better to take the vaccine before the epidemic, not during it.

This was different in that it surprised us, and no vaccine was available. It also appeared to induce an increased death rate than the usual influenza virus. Many were hospitalized, although the treatment was usually only supportive therapy.

A new type of vaccine was created to treat this new, non-influenza virus. It was important in that this was not an influenza vaccine. Our immune system had little recognition of a virus like this in the past and hence could not mount an efficient adaptive immune response. I will discuss vaccines in a later chapter.

This new type of vaccine could be developed rapidly, and it was. I say new, but vaccines of this type had been in the process of development, just not used on a large population of humans. An experimental vaccine was approved without the usually waiting time for a normal vaccine. This was then given to a large portion of the US and the rest of the world. At the time of my writing this. about 85% of adults in the US have gotten this vaccine.

This time period is fresh in my memory and although this was not a perfect solution, if was better than nothing. I would have done the same thing if I were in control.

That was $2^1/_2$ years ago, and we know a lot more about the virus and the vaccine today. This book is about Covid, the vaccine, and our health, in the context of the paper I have referenced.

I read this paper numerous times. It is not a particularly easy read and I had to look up several topics during the reading to get an understanding of his explanations and predictions. I now have a pretty good idea of the conclusions but have discovered it is extremely difficult to adequately explain it to the common man. As I have noted in all my books, it is not that the common man is not capable of reasoning it out, it is just that most do not understand the language of the science.

My job is to teach you the language so that you can use your common sense to arrive at a conclusion. I will explain what the author's conclusion is, but do not think that this is necessarily my conclusion.

Like many other health decisions the government has made in the past, some I do not agree with. My beef is with the government, not with any particular political party and I hope to keep politics out of the discussion. I will disagree with many of the government's policies in this book, but that is not to say I may not have done the same thing, just implemented it a lot differently.

Unlike previous epidemics, the press and social media have played a large role in how the virus, the vaccine, the government actions, and our health has been presented. I am going to give you enough information to understand the paper and let you come to your own decisions. At the end I will tell you what I believe regarding health and covid, the governmental decisions regarding this epidemic, and the advice I give family and friends.

I am not practicing medicine; therefore, I do not have to worry about the medical board, governmental agencies, bosses, being sued, an employer, the FBI, or being banned by social media. I also do not have to worry about being called stupid or crazy as that has already happened numerous times. I do want you to be able to evaluate what you hear, see on TV, or read about and make up your own mind using your common sense.

The next few chapters are to remind you what you may have learned in college years ago, but since hardly anyone uses this information routinely, you may have forgotten it. Some of you may never have learned it. In any case, look through it and it will begin to sound familiar.

VIRUS

Some of you recall my other books. Before I could explain diabetes, I had to explain carbs, fats, and protein. Before I could explain eating, I had to teach you about metabolism. Finally, we could talk about diet.

This is a book about Covid Vaccines and Health. To start with I need to give you some basics about viruses. You will recall that before I could teach you about epigenetics, I had to review the basics of cell biology and DNA. I am going to do the same thing now with viruses. Eventually when I write about epigenetics and the gut biome, I am going to teach you about bacteria.

First naming. Viruses are named based upon similarities in their structure and organization of their genotype. The virus we are interested in is a member of the family coronavirus. This is the family from which most of the common cold viruses arrive. This is usually an upper respiratory tract infection.

Covid is the name of the illness caused by this virus, just as influenza is the name of an illness caused by a virus in the orthomyxovirus family.

The designation of this virus is SARS-CoV-2. This is because there was an outbreak of sudden acute respiratory disease in the middle east in 2003. This was a coronavirus and was designated SARS-CoV-1 which stands for Severe Acute Respiratory Syndrome Coronavirus. The current covid disease virus is very similar in structure to this virus hence the name SARS-Cov-2

It is also called Covid-19 which stands for coronavirus disease of 2019. In this book when I say covid, I will mean either the virus or the disease, you should be able to tell by the context or I will make it clear to you.

When I taught you about cell biology, there were many different organelles required to make everything in the cell. Remember the cell has the capacity to make all its structures, in other words, to make a new cell. It does this all the time.

A virus has four structures for the most part. It has a core of RNA or DNA made of nucleic acids and protein, it has a coating around this made of protein called a capsid, some have a lipid coating called an envelope, and then there is a protein on the outside which enables the virus to attach to a cell via a receptor.

All of these elements were made by some host cell. The virus cannot make anything on its own. It infects a cell, then induces the cell to make a bunch more viruses which are called virions.

This is the basic virus. Some can insert their DNA into yours and be passed onto the next generation. Some can remain dormant in a cell for years, they have different shapes and different ways of getting into the cell, but all have in common that they cannot make anything for themselves.

Now I am going to confine the discussion to the covid virus. This may be a little detailed but keep reading it till you understand. You need to learn the language of this virus to understand the vaccines.

Remember the point of this book is to enable you to understand the science in the paper written by Dr. G Vanden Bossche so you can use your common sense to see what you think about the conclusions.

I of course will tell you what I think at the end, but you will need to read the book to be able to understand that.

By now everyone has seen a picture of this virus. This is a statement I would never have believed I could make 20 years ago. And I mean an actual picture, not just an artist's conception. It does look a little blurry, but it is amazing we can see this.

With computer assistance we can see an extremely accurate picture of the whole virus in great detail, including the structure of the protein and even individual molecules. These appear to be quite accurate.

We see a ball with projections extending out about a fourth of the diameter long. There are 25 to 40 of these projections which are made from protein. They appear to be bushy at the top and skinnier at the bottom where they attach to the body of the virus. This is composed of three copies of a protein called the spike protein (although it looks more like a stalk). At the top each protein is an enlarged area which contains the area where the spike initially connects to the host cell. This is called the receptor binding domain on the spike protein.

Since the spike is composed of three proteins (the same ones), there are three of these receptor binding domains on each spike. If you looked down upon this spike structure it would look like a tulip with three petals. These petals can be in a position in which they are open or closed. The other end of the spike is where the virus is attached to the body of the virus. When a petal is open, it can attach to a receptor on the host cell which we can visualize as a small petal which matches up to the tulip petal.

Now I need you to use your imagination to get an idea of the size. Let's say a cell is about the size of a nice smooth basketball. If we looked at a virion on the ball, we would see the spike protein to appear be as long as one day's growth of a beard on the basketball (.3mm) and the virion body to be about the size of a mustard seed. We would not be able to see the stalk because it would be way too skinny, but we might be able to feel it if you rubbed your hand across it. In real life you would not because it is too thin to feel. The receptor on the ball is only about a fourth of the size of the spike so, even though there may be more than 100,000 spread around the surface of the ball, you would not see or feel them. One glucose molecule is 1/30 the size of the spike protein so of course you could not see that either. You may wonder how a mustard seed can take over a basketball. Well, a normal mustard seed can grow almost to the size of a basketball in about six weeks.

Back to normal size. Many of you recall Brownian motion, which is the random motion of small particles suspended in liquid or gas. Many of us have looked through a microscope and seen bacteria wiggling around. This is due to the collision of water molecules.

If you have a cell in a liquid, it is constantly being bombarded by small particles. These could be glucose molecules, bacteria, chylomicrons, proteins of all types, or virions. Things are bouncing off the cell wall all the time which excludes them unless there is a receptor there whereby the particle binds to a receptor which activates a chemical reaction, often mediated by an enzyme, which permits the particle to enter through a pore or engulfed by a vacuole budding into the cell membrane.

Virions are often bouncing off the cell membrane. The spike protein is wiggling all over the place. And the receptors on the cell wall are moving around. Randomly one of these spikes can get very close to the cell receptor and a transient chemical bond can form. This often triggers a reaction from the cell membrane. such that chemical changes occur in the membrane.

There are many different types of receptors on the cell, and the receptors often bind numerous different substances. Of course, the cell does not have a covid receptor, but the virus is able to bind to a ACE2 receptor which is found in the respiratory tract among other places (ACE is angiotensin converting enzyme) This is the same place the SARS Cov-1 virus bind to, but the covid virus is much better at it.

Once the stalk binds to the receptor, numerous changes take place The spike protein has two subunits named site 1 and site 2. Site one is the part which contains the area that binds the receptor. When the surface protease is activated, it cuts a segment on site 2 which exposes several hydrophobic amino acids. Hydrophobic means it doesn't like water. When these are exposed, water and Brownian motion pushes these toward the fatty cell surface and the amino acids embed themselves and attach the body to the cell membrane.

Iin other words, a portion of the top part of this spike protein binds to the cell, and a chemical process occurs such that the bottom half of the spike protein binds such that the rest of the body of the virus draws closer to the surface of the cell.

This hinge site is sometimes referred to as the furin site, furin referring to a group or protease enzymes. The snipping of the amino acids at this site increases the infectivity of the virus. SARS has this site, but it only contains one amino acid. Covid virus has five amino acids at this hinge site and snipping these increases the infectivity. Some believe that if you were modifying the coronavirus to become more virulent, this is where you would insert amino acids.

You can imagine that activating the furin site causes stalk protein to bend and hence draw the virus body closer to the cell surface such that it may contact the cell surface and activate the surface to engulf the virus, which then enters the cell and begins the process to induce the cell to begin making more viruses. That is infect the cell.

The old spike (unit 1) is then not needed. It has already done its job of attaching to the receptor and activating the process of entering the cell. Unit 1 may then separate and travel elsewhere and cause other problems as it still has the ability to interact with a receptor. There are new amino acid "spikes" which come out of unit 2 which merge to the cell membrane and begin to fold and bring the body of the virion down along the hinge between unit 1 and unit 2. When the body of the virion lands on the cell membrane, further enzymes are activated which allows the virion to merge with the cell. The mustard seed is now inside.

If the virus enters the cell through the receptor, the viral membrane merges with the cell membrane and just the mRNA is injected.

Turns out the virion can alternatively be engulfed by the cell membrane in a vacuole, without going through the receptor. In that case a different enzyme is activated when the virion lands on the cell. This process is not as efficient but is the main pathway with the SARS-1 virus. In this case the whole virion is inside the cell. The different variants may have slightly different mechanisms and amino acids that change this slightly.

Once inside it is more difficult to stop the virus. You can see it would be easiest just to keep the virus from binding to the receptor, and that is what the adaptive immune system does. Once in, the immune system takes care of this just by destroying the cell. Your immune system does not have access to the virus once it is in the cell. You make millions of cells every day, so you won't miss it.

The protein spike has done its job and is discarded. The envelope of the virus is gone and now we have the RNA inside. If you recall my book, *Introduction to Cell Biology and Epigenetics*, this RNA is mRNA and will go to the ribosome to begin making more proteins. The RNA has about 30,000 base pairs (half that since this is a single strand RNA) which translates into about 5 miles using my illustration of the DNA ladder with base pairs being one foot apart. One normal human chromosome is 28,000 miles which is around the world. This RNA codes for 29 different proteins. The virion had proteins (enzymes) available when it entered the cells that were produced by its previous host cell. The enzymes present and the new enzymes from the mRNA take over the cell in various ways. It eliminates any mRNA that is not tagged as viral, it markedly reduces overall mRNA transcription by plugging up the pores in the nuclear membrane through with the mRNA normally passes, and what transcription (changing mRNA to protein) occurs is confined to making new virions. It also prevents mRNA from leaving the nucleus such that interferon in not produced which would alert the immune system that something is wrong here. Your body has various mechanisms by which it can recognize the infected cell is abnormal and kill the virus, now within the cell, by just destroying the whole cell.

The virus now starts its crusade to take over the cell and produce virions. It is estimated that an infected person produces 1-10 billion virions a day, with an infected cell producing up to one million virions a day at the peak of infection We can try to keep the virus from entering the cell, we can try to delay its production, we can try to keep the virions from being released, and finally we can just get rid of the cell.

The numbers have been carefully examined: and appear to be valid estimates.

The mRNA produces lots of copies of itself. There is a complicated process to convert these copies into infectious units. It has been calculated that 10,000 virions need to be produced to make one infections unit. Hence' we end up with 100 infectious units per infected cell at peak production which lasts 1-3 days) per cell.

Many copies of RNA are produced in the cell. An infectious unit is the completely encapsulated virus released by the cell ready to infect which is a much lower number than virions. if we say 10, infectious units are produced by each infected cell a day, we can calculate that there are about a million infected cells per person, most all of these in the lung.

Overall, it is estimated that the total number of infectious units over the complete course of an infection is $3 \times 10^5 - 3 \times 10^8$.

I talked about the ACE2 receptor as the entry of the virus into the cell. Less than 10% of lung cells have this receptor (about 10^9 cells). The total number of infected cells in the lung is about 10^5. Therefore, only about 1 in 10,00 of the available lung cells get infected.

So far, most people agree with all I have told you. That will not be true of the whole book. Like everyone else. I must rely on the information from others. It is nice if everyone agrees. Everyone does not agree with Dr. Bossche's paper. Now a little background on immunology.

The infection produced 10 billion virions (10^{11}) ; you have 3×10^{13} cells in your body. Therefore, the cells outnumber the virions more than 100 to 1.

IMMUNOLOGY

Most of us have a general understanding of the immune system. We know that it prevents, or fights infections caused by microbes, which is bacteria, viruses, fungi, or parasites. Basically, anything that does not belong to you. We also know that this process can go amiss and start attacking things that are you. This is an autoimmune disease.

The immune system is quite complicated, but I am not going to teach you everything about it. We need to learn about two aspects of this system, which is the innate system and the acquired system. The innate system is on call all the time, while the acquired system responds to pathogens we have seen before or look like things we have seen before.

I am going to teach you about the covid virus and covid vaccine, but much applies to any virus or vaccine. It would be easier if we all had the same functioning system, but we don't. I guess I should not say that. We have the same system, but it does not work the same for everyone.

If you are under six months old, you have not developed your own system yet. Eventually you do and are like everyone else. If you are in poor health due to wearing out, poor lifetime diet, accumulated expose to unhealthy aspects of the environment, or perhaps a genetic aspect, then your immune system does not work as well (immunosenescence) . As you age, lots of systems don't work as well.

You could be on the other end and your immune system is hyperactive. That is, it starts destroying your own cells and you have autoimmune disease. Or maybe just hayfever

At this point everyone knows this, and I am not telling you anything new. We all know covid has a much higher death rate in old people or people in poor health. It really is not necessarily that you are old as many old people are in good health, it is rather that we have decided to use age as a marker of health. You are more likely to die of covid if you are old and perhaps in poor health, but not if you are old and in good health. (That is if I am comparing you to other old people. No matter how good your health is, if you are old, you still have a greater chance of dying than a normal young person) I am going stick to the immune system.

There is another category of people at greater risk. That is those who have elevated blood sugar (Diabetes, Prediabetes, obesity).

There are some people who have poor immune systems because we are giving them medication that depresses the immune system. People with autoimmune disease or cancer treatment or some who just have a poor system for some other reasons. In many of these we have determined that it is better for us to treat the condition, which may then depress the immune system, rather than let the disease progress. The treatment may make you feel better than if we did nothing, but you do have a greater risk of dying from covid.

For the most part, the statistic I am concerned with is dying from covid. The number of covid cases is a soft statistic. We can say how many have a positive test, but we know many do not get tested in the first place. If you have a mild case or perhaps you don't like to go to the doctor or maybe it costs money and time and you just stay home, then we don't know how many cases there are. Still the number of positive cases gives us baseline, otherwise like the current epidemic, anyone who does not feel well will claim they have covid.

We also look at the number of hospitalizations. This statistic is easier to find, and we can assume you do not get put in the hospital for covid unless you have a positive test. Poor people and people without insurance do not get put in the hospital as much. In many countries there may not be enough hospitals, or you may not be able to afford them. Still, it is not a bad statistic and gives us a pretty good idea of the risk of getting covid.

I now am using the chart which shows hospital admissions as a marker of covid infections since now that the cases are so mild, no one gets a test or reports it anywhere. Admissions will give us a better idea as to the rising or falling incidence of infections.

Finally, we have death. This is a good statistic as it is objective. Every modern country with a functioning government usually keeps track of the number of deaths. Someone writes it down if you die. Most countries have kept track of this statistic for many years, sometimes a couple hundred years. We know if you die, but did you die of covid? With the current epidemic the question always arises; did you die of covid or with covid? We know the covid deaths have been overstated somewhat as there is just too much to gain by claiming covid was the cause of death. By that I mean someone gets paid more. This may not be as true in some countries that don't give the hospital or patient a bonus if they die of covid, yet still this is a good statistic to follow. I may not know for sure if you died of covid, but I do know you died of something, and it was accurately recorded.(We estimate based upon examination of medical records that about 30% of covid deaths are those who died with covid, not from covid (at least in the USA)

There is an excess death statistic: that is, you take the average number of deaths in the past few years before covid, subtract the number of real covid deaths, and you get more or less of the average number of deaths. If more, these ae the excess deaths for that year. Simply more deaths than you would expect).

This statistic has gathered much interest in the past few months. Now that the vaccine has been around almost three years, different countries have analyzed data that makes it appear there have been more deaths than expected, even after you eliminate the covid deaths which we believed are too high to begin with (recall the problems of dying of covid and dying with covid) These deaths with but not of covid are believed to make the death rate from covid to be 10-20% higher than it really is. Even using the inflated covid death rate, it appears there are still 15-20% more deaths than we would have predicted. This is substantiated by private industry when looking at the insurance payments for death claims.

Back to the immune system. We are going to divide the immune responses into two systems, the innate immune system, and the adaptive system. Innate means you were born with this system. The adaptive system develops throughout your life.

The innate system is always on call and is the immediate response system for anything unwanted that is able to enter your body through the skin barrier. The barrier separates the outside from your inside. Of course, the skin is the main barrier, but your gut lining is also separating outside from inside. Before you get to the stomach, we have the mucous lining of the nasopharynx, mouth, throat, and esophagus. Your eyes can be an entry point, as can the urethra. These are all lined by different types of cells.

Once penetrated, certain cells in your system respond. These cells are white blood cells and come in several types. This group of cells are also called granulocytes in that they are full of what appear to be granules which are specialized vacuoles in the cell that contain various enzymes, chemicals, and messenger cells that can either be released, or used to digest particles these cells may have ingested.

Neutrophils are the most abundant white cells and are the first responders. These cells are able to engulf foreign particles and destroy them. These cells also ingest dead parts of other cellular materials and can then recycle some of the amino acids.

There are also basophils, which can ingest allergens , and eosinophils who are responsible for attacking parasites. Mast cells are also a part of this system and release histamine which promotes inflammation.

All these cells contain many receptors on the cell surface in order to determine if this particle is part of you and hence, we should leave it alone, or foreign and we should eliminate it. These receptors are generalized such that they may recognize a lipopolysaccharide that is common to bacteria and phagocytize it, while the adaptive system which makes antibodies is quite particular as to what these antibodies attack. For our interest the white blood cells can recognize and engulf viruses . As we will see later, it is much easier for them to do this if there are antibodies attached to the particle. If an antibody is attached, that signals the white cell to engulf it.

These cells are important in that they release some of these granules when they begin identifying foreign matter which causes inflammation. The chemicals attract other white blood cells to the area as well as dilate the blood vessels and allow more cells to leave the circulation and enter the tissue. We see this as swelling, redness, and soreness from these chemicals.

This system is working all the time. These cells can also identify cells that are broken or infected and destroy the cells and all their contents.

A part of the innate system is interferon which is made by almost all the cells. Interferon is activated when a cell is invaded by a virus. This interferon can then communicate with neighboring cells such that they will try to prevent virus entry and replication within the neighbor cell. This interferon also causes the infected cells to undergo apoptosis, which is natural cell destruction. The treatment of a viral infected cell is to kill the cell and destroy its contents. Once the cell has been infected it cannot be cured and must be destroyed. More so, the body does what it can to prevent the cell from infecting other cells.

We want to identify a virus when it invades, we then want to destroy the cell that has been infected, we then want to prevent infection to other cells. Interferon is an important group of chemicals that help destroy infected cells and tries to stimulate other cells not to get infected.

Another component of the innate system is the compliment system. These are a group of proteins present in the blood in an inactive state. Inflammation attracts these proteins to the site and as the components are in one place, there is a series of reactions in which one protein activates the next stage to produce a protein that activates the next stage and so on. When you get to the end you have cytotoxic chemicals that directly destroy cells by affecting the cell membrane. These are potent chemicals, and you do not what to activate them by accident, hence you must go through a cascade to get them to work.

Again, the cell gets infected by a virus, you can't cure it, you must destroy it. At the same time, you don't want to go around destroying perfectly normal cells. Once sensitized to a specific antigen, IgG can prevent infection by binding to the virus before it infects the cell. Once it has attached to an antigen on the virus, this signals the other cells to engulf or kill this virus. The same thing happens when the antibodies attach to an infected cell. It signals the other cells in the immune system to destroy this cell.

Once the IgG producing cells are activated, large quantities of the antibodies are produced making sure all the antigens are tagged and destroyed. The antibodies themselves to not destroy the virus/cells, rather it gets other cells to do it.

The IgG can interfere with the binding and entry of the virus into the cell, but once in, it can only notify others that this cell is infected.

Covid, and other viruses, attempt to evade the innate immunes system by using glycosides similar to what the body uses to identify yourself from something else. Once inside the cell, one of the first jobs of the mRNA is to make proteins which inhibit the cell from making interferon. Your adaptive immune system's job is to keep the virus from infecting the cell, and if that fails, identify this cell as infected so your innate immune system can destroy the cell.

To complete the innate system cells we have everyone's favorite, which is the NK cells or natural killer cells. These are not white blood cells but lymphocytes. They are always present in the blood and comprise up to 20% of the lymphocytes. They go around looking for cells that don't belong. If you get a viral infection, you decrease the MHC or major histocompatibility complex which is on the cell surface. If you do not have that, the NK cells destroy that cell by the use of chemicals which induces the cell to destroy itself. A viral infection changes these MHCs and thus also flags this cell to be the target of the NK cell. It ends up tumors also do not express the right MHC and the NK cells participate in preventing cancers.

I should make this a little clearer. NK cells do not engulf cells. They primarily kill cells by activating apoptosis in the cell. In other words, the cell kills itself. They can also release granules that disrupt the cell membrane and allow the outside environment to pour in. More granules get in and more water and thus you get osmotic cell lysis. The NK cells can also recognize antibodies that may be attached to the cell which activate the NK cell to destroy that cell. Later I will talk about the activated cytotoxic lymphocytes. They are a lot like the NK cell but are directed to only destroy cells displaying a certain antigen, like antibodies which only attach to specific antigens. The NK cells are not as picky as the cytotoxic lymphocytes and are attracted to general types of antigens.

The WBCs can release chemicals that attract these NK cells, thus in the presence of inflammation, induced by the WBCs, there are plenty of these NK cells around. When the cells get destroyed by the NK cell, the neutrophils can then engulf these cellular parts. In a minute I will talk about the adaptive immune system which involves different kinds of lymphocytes.

There are three more neutrophils that we need to know about.

Monocytes, which are part of the innate system, mainly reside in the blood. When the enter the tissue, they are called **macrophages**. These are the largest phagocytic cells. The other neutrophil is the **dendritic cell**. They also can phagocytize things. These cells are the connection between the innate system and the adaptive system.

These cells can engulf a virus, a bacterium, or other small foreign object. They can then digest these particles into packets containing around 10 amino acids. They then take these packets to the cell surface attached to MHC 2 , the major histocompatibility complex, which is .a group of proteins. This MHC group of proteins transport the packet filled with the `10 amino acids to the surface of the cell. Lymphocytes then can recognize these packets and eventually antibodies are formed to this packet of amino acids. The innate system is not very specific and just recognizes general categories. An antibody which is part of the adaptive system is quite specific to these amino acids and can sometimes differentiate between a particle with only one amino acid difference. These cells, the monocytes, macrophages and dendritic cells, are called antigen presenting cells as they signal the system to begin making antibodies to this particular antigen by presenting them to the lymph nodes.

The dendritic cell is an antigen presenting cell and can travel around in the body. Once they engulf antigens, they become activated and usually can travel to various lymph nodes or the spleen (as well as other areas) in order to present these antigens to the families of lymphocytes residing there. It ends up these are important to our study of covid and vaccines. I will talk more about them next.

The innate system is always on call and very efficient in destroying invaders. For a time, we did not consider them to have a memory. The adaptive system creates memory cells that linger for years and jump into action if that antigen is recognized at a later date. The innate system had cells that recognized general antigens, but not specific ones like the adaptive system. We now recognize . there can be training of the innate system which acts somewhat like adaptive memory cells. I will discuss this later.

Finally, we have IgM, an antibody that is considered part of the innate system. In the adaptive system, the antibodies are highly specific. The IgM antibodies have a much wider range of antigens to which they can bind. These can then activate the compliment cascade and cause cell death. IgM is always hanging around in the tissue and blood looking for general categories of antigens to which it can bind.

The second half of our immune system is the adaptive system. This means that as time goes on its sensitivities change. This is the system that enables vaccines to perform. For a vaccine, antigens are administered to the body (vaccine shot) and the body produces antibodies to those antigens. Memory cells are created such that if those antigens can be recognized in the future, and your body can rapidly remake antibodies to these antigens. It takes several weeks before your body processes a new antigen and generate cells that produce IgG against that antigen. The next time it is exposed it only takes a few days to start the IgG flowing.

That is the way vaccines work. You get sensitized to a specific antigen which may take a few weeks, your antibody production is suddenly elevated, and if you recognize that antigen again a few years later, you already have cells around that can make that specific antibody hence the response is much more rapid.

A few details how this works. This system is made up of two different lymphocytes. The B cells are the ones involved in making antibodies. The other half is the T cells which are involved in cell mediated immunity, which means they identify cells with this antigen and kill it. Both have memory cells.

This means you have cells which are already sensitized to a specific antigen, and they can reactivate to rapidly produce antibodies, and different lymphocytes which have also been sensitized to this antigen, which can begin rapidly reproducing and generate cytotoxic lymphocytes which destroy the cells expressing this antigen.

The T cells are divided into **helper T cells** and **cytotoxic T cells.** The helper cells are also called **CD4** cells, and the cytotoxic are called **CD8** cells. When these cells are initially formed in your bone marrow, they are naïve. That means they are not sensitized to any particular antigen. They must be primed by exposure to be able to begin reproducing.

Before I go on, let me review. Your body gets infected, either by bacteria or a virus. The macrophages and dendritic cells are particularly present at the boundary between outside and inside. For covid it is in the upper respiratory tract that the virus enters. It will encounter a macrophage or a dendritic cell. These cells have receptors that will recognize this foreign body as not-self and will engulf the pathogen. Inside the cell the pathogen is encased in a vacuole and partially digested into amino acid segments, around 10 to 20 amino acids in length. These are then attached to one of the **MHC-2** (major histocompatibility complexes) and transported to the cell membrane. The T cell lymphocyte (in the lymph node) can then recognize the antigen and if it is the correct antigen, that is the antigen the cell was created to recognize, attaches to this antigen and becomes activated.

The macrophage is local, whereas the dendritic cell does the same thing but travels to the lymph nodes where it presents these antigens to naive B cells and T cells. There are lots of different naïve B cells with antibodies directed at many different antigens. When the right B cell finds the correct presented antigen. It becomes partially activated and when fully activated can start reproducing. The naïve T cells have receptors, but like the B cells, each one is only sensitive to one antigen, and once the right one is found, it binds to this antigen and the T cell is activated. Each naïve T cell only has one antigen which will activate it.

The dendritic cell travels around presenting this antigen on its surface attached to the MHC to lymphocytes in the lymph nodes. If a memory lymphocyte recognizes this antigen, it goes into action making antibodies. If a naïve B lymphocyte, meaning a cell formed in the marrow to recognize this antigen but has never been activated, recognizes this antigen on the dendrite cell, it becomes partially activated and can subsequently become fully activated with a helper T cell.

Once a B cell is activated, usually through interaction with an activated T-helper cell, the B cell begins rapidly dividing. Some turn into plasma cells which make antibodies against this antigen, and some turn into memory cells that can last a long time such that if this antigen is recognized in the future, it can immediately start dividing and making more antibodies.

The same thing will happen to the T cell in the lymph node They have receptors attached to the cell membrane which, when the correct antigen gets attached, will be activated, and begin dividing.

The T cells are divided into T helper cells (CD 4 cells) and cytotoxic T cells (CD-8) There are naïve cytotoxic CD-8 cells floating around in your body as well as in your lymph nodes. If you have a cell in your body which is infected with covid (or any bacteria or virus), this particle can be digested in the cells and pieces about 10 amino acids long can be attached to an **MHC-1** carrier and then travel to the cell membrane and be exposed on the **MCH-1** carrier to the outside. A T-cell (CD-8) with the right receptor can then bind with this antigen and become activated.

The Dendritic cell attaches the antigen to the MHC 2 complex which subsequently gets exposed to correct naïve B cells in the lymph node, and with the help of the right helper T lymphocyte can eventually activate the B cell to make antibodies.

A naïve cytotoxic T lymphocyte floating around in your body can eventually interact with the antigen it was formed to recognize attached to the surface of and infected cell by the MHC 1 group of proteins and become activated.

This cell will then travel to the lymph node and begin reproducing itself. The cells reproduced will either be a cytotoxic T cell against that antigen, or a memory T cell which may be around for years waiting for that antigen to reappear so it can begin reproducing again. Meanwhile the primed cytotoxic T cell goes around destroying cells expressing this antigen. When a cell is infected with covid, or any virus, antigens are expressed on the cell surface which can be recognized by the sensitized cytotoxic T cell (CD 8). The cytotoxic T cell can then destroy the cell marked with this antigen.

The T helper cells, the CD 4 cells, go around completing the activating the naïve B cells, which we activated by recognizing the antigen attached to the MHC-2 complex, for which this cell was formed to recognize. With the help of the right T cell (CD 4) attached to the partially activated B cell, which also recognized the correct antigen, the B cell can start creating antibodies.

To be clear, macrophages and dendritic cells can engulf viruses, digest them, and attach small parts of them to **MHC-2** complexes which present these antigens on the cell membrane. All cells which become infected with a virus can attach pieces of this virus (antigens) to **MHC-1** complexes on the cell membrane. If a dendritic cell gets infected, it will also present pieces of the virus on MHC-1 complexes along with the pieces of viruses it engulfed and subsequently attached to the **MHC-2** complexes.

The dendritic cell travels to the lymph node and throughout the body. It possesses antigens attached to MHC complexes (**both MHC-1 and MHC-2**) and can also have whole virions attached to the cell membrane by a different mechanism. The antigens are presented to naïve T helper CD 4 cells which recognize the MHC-2 protein and can attach to the antigen. Again, you have millions of naïve helper T cells in the lymph node each one which may be recognizing a different antigen. The one with the right receptor recognizes this antigen. These activated T cells can also recognize antigens in the tissue even if they are not attached to antigen presenting cells.

CD4 stands for cluster of differentiation 4 and is a glycoprotein we use to identify certain cells. For our purposes, T helper cells , monocytes, macrophages, and dendritic cells are CD4 cells and are involved with MHC-2 complexes.

The naïve cytotoxic CD-8 lymphocytes are going around looking at MCH-1 complexes trying to find the antigen that matches its assigned antigen, and if found, becomes an activated cytotoxic lymphocyte which will start reproducing and forming other cytotoxic lymphocytes that will seek to destroy any cells presenting this antigen. It will also form memory cytotoxic lymphocytes.

When the helper CD-4 T cell recognizes its antigen on the MHC-2 and becomes activated, it begins reproducing into a memory cell that begin excreting cytokines (chemicals that enhance inflammation) and attract other cells to the inflammatory site upon recognition of the antigen. It also will go to the lymph node where the dendritic cell is presenting this antigen so that it can attach to the B-cell presenting this same antigen and activate the B cell This will cause reproduction of the activated cells which will turn into another memory cell, and into plasma cells which will begin producing loads of antibodies.

You are born with some of your innate immune system already sensitized to certain pathogens. You also want your immune system to be able to differentiate between you and something else. Sometimes between you and another person. As you get older your immune systems memory expands. Sometimes it begins reacting to a disease you have not had before, but it is close enough to another disease that it reacts.

Once the innate immune system recognizes abnormal structures or cells, chemical messaging attracts different cells to the site. All of us are familiar with white blood cells, which are leukocytes. These cells engulf pathogens or other cells by killing them. When you get a CBC, we will measure the level of white cells. If they are elevated, you may have an infection. These cells are often marginated in the blood vessels, which means they are on the walls. When signaled they then enter the stream and go to the site. The CBC counts the number that are in the liquid part of the blood.

Antibodies are made by the B lymphocytes. Once a lymphocyte has been activated to secrete a specific antibody, it will always secrete that one. If more antibody is needed, the lymphocyte will begin reproducing and all the offspring will produce the same antibody. All of them will be the same and hence monoclonal. You can have a node with several different lymphocytes producing different antibodies and hence are polyclonal.

Let us review. The T cells recognize antigens on the cell surface of the cell. If the cell gets infected with a virus or bacteria, some of the proteins are transferred to the cell wall by the major histocompatibility molecules (MHM) You do not make antibodies against the entire virus, but rather to a small piece of a protein in the virus, around 10 -15 amino acids long. The antibodies you make are very specific and may be able to differentiate between segments that only differ by one amino acid. So, you make several different antibodies against the same virus, all against different segments of proteins. In addition, this protein segment may be common to other proteins such that the antibody may attach to several different proteins that happen to contain this same peptide segment.

The T lymphocytes recognize these antigens when they are part of the histocompatibility complex, and some (**the CD-8** who are looking at **MHC-1 complexes** then turn into cytotoxic T cells. Some ,the **CD-4 helper T lymphocytes** who are looking for antigens attached **to MHC-2 complexes**, can become activated by finding the correct antigen and can then activate B lymphocytes to start making antibodies. The B lymphocytes can also engulf antigens, attach histocompatibility complexes (MHC-2), and present these to T helper cells, so that the B cell becomes activated when the T cell with that antigen attaches to it. The B lymphocytes eventually turn into plasma cells, reproduce, and make antibodies. Along the way some of these turn into memory cells that will start this process again if it recognizes this antigen in the future. For a B cell to become activated, it must come into contact with the specific antigen it is programmed to react to, either by engulfing the antigen or attaching to a dendritic cell presenting the antigen, and then must also interact with an activated CD-4 T cell which also has become activated by coming into contact with that specific antigen.

Infected cells present antigens on MHC-1` complexes. . Macrophages can engulf pathogens, digest them, attach the parts to histocompatibility complexes, both on MHC-1 and MHC-2 complexes, and present them to the surface such that the T cells can recognize them. At the same time this is happening many different chemicals are released that dilate blood vessels and attract various other cells hence we get inflammation.

The dendritic cells are more motile and can engulf antigens, attach them for presentation. They can also attach the whole virions to the cell membrane, and then travel to lymph nodes or the spleen to present these antigens to lymphocytes. It turns out that these cells can attach the virion without breaking it down into antigens The virion is tethered to the outside of the dendritic cell membrane. This virion is still intact and if transported somewhere else, can infect a cell in that neighborhood.

For our purposes with covid and vaccines, we are interested in the antibody attaching to the pathogen to prevent infection. Antibodies have other uses such as attaching to cells to stimulate their destruction or attaching to toxins to prevent their entering the cell or attaching to pathogens such that they are engulfed and destroyed. In case of a viral or bacterial infection, antibodies can also prevent cell to cell spread of these pathogens.

Covid invades through the mucosa in the upper respiratory tract. Antibodies, especially IgA, which is found in mucus, can attach to pathogens, and cause them to agglutinate and be eliminated from the body through the mucus. Either coughing, spitting, or swallowing the mucous to the acid stomach will remove pathogens.

The central issue in this book as far as antibodies are concerned revolves around antibody production that would prevent an infection with covid. The mechanism of interest is to prevent the attachment of the covid virion spike protein to the cell by blocking the receptor on the spike and preventing attachment to the ACE2 receptor.

It is possible I have not explained this well enough, so I am going to present another mental image of this process.

Lymphocytes are made in the bone marrow as immature cells with no receptors. Your body then creates many different types of receptors to replicate all the different antigens that you could possibly encounter. It attaches a different one to each lymphocyte. You can image this to be like membrane bound antibodies attached to the cell surface. They do not leave the surface to attach themselves to particles floating around, but if they encounter this antigen, and each cell only has one type, it will activate that cell.

There appears to be about 10 billion possible antigenic combinations which means at least 10 billion different lymphocytes. First your body must remove the lymphocytes that have antigens which are normally present in your body so that you do not develop antibodies against yourself or cytotoxic t cells that will attack you. Then you have billions of the rest of these lymphocytes floating around in your body, each one with a different antigen Now there are more than one lymphocyte per antigen floating around, but still each lymphocyte has only one type of antigen. As you can imagine, most may never get used for anything. These cells remain naïve.

We have naïve B lymphocytes, Helper T lymphocytes, and cytotoxic lymphocytes floating around looking for the right antigens. I say floating around, but many naïve lymphocytes are found in lymph nodes or the spleen.

Now let us look at all the nucleated cells in your body, which is most of them. All of these cells produce MHC-1 complexes in themselves which are continually presenting antigens to the surface of the cell. These are antigens found in the cell. They do not have to be from infections or even foreign antigens. This is simply so the immune system can recognize the cell and make sure it is a normal antigen that is supposed to be there. Recall the quality control system in your body is always identifying abnormal proteins which it then digests into 10-20 amino acid sized antigens which it then attaches to MHC complexes and is then displayed on the surface of the cell. This is always going on in the cell and if the cell is the size of a basketball, these complexes are about the size of a period.

The naïve cytotoxic lymphocytes are looking around for these MHC-1 complexes which may be displaying the antigen that activates them. If they finally find their antigen on the MHC-1 on a cell, the lymphocyte will become activated. It will then begin reproducing and making more cytotoxic lymphocytes, as well as some memory cytotoxic lymphocytes, which will then destroy the cells expressing this antigen. This antigen could be coming from a viral infection, a bacterial infection, or a cancer cell, basically anything making a protein not native to the cell which the cell as subsequently presented an MHC-1 complex. When the cell is infected with covid, many virions, up to a billion a day, are being manufactured. About one in 10,00 of them are being transported to the cell membrane in order to be released into fluid surrounding our cells. The cell is also displaying pieces of the virus to the cell membrane on MHC-1 complexes which the immune system can recognize.

As long has the antigens are around you make more cytotoxic lymphocytes to that antigen. Eventually you win and the antigen goes away, but just in case you now have memory cells with this antigen floating around. In other words, you have more of these lymphocytes with this antigen looking for this antigen than you had before, and hence you get a more rapid response if the antigen re-appears.

A bunch of other things happen when the lymphocyte gets activated as all kinds of cytokines and interferon is released which enhances the immune response.

Now we have the remaining helper T cells and B cells. They also have their singular antigen and are floating around. Some are just hanging around in lymph nodes. They are looking for antigens attached to the MHC 2 complex. All cells, including these naïve lymphocytes, have MHC 1 complexes. Only a few cells have the ability to express antigens on the MHC-2 complex. These cells are the B lymphocytes, the macrophages, and the dendritic cells.

MHC-1 antigens come from within the cell. This could be an abnormal protein the cell made or was infected with. MHC-2 antigens come from without the cells. In other words, the antigen on the MHC-2 came from a particle which the presenting cells has engulfed. A covid virion can infect a cell and be presented on an MHC-1 which a cytotoxic lymphocyte can use to become activated, or it can be ingested by the dendritic cell, macrophage, or B cell and be presented on an MHC-2 which will activate the B cell or helper T cell, and hence result in antibody formation.

Macrophages and dendritic cells have this ability to engulf, digest and present. These two cells are often hanging around the boundaries of the body looking for things which may have gotten in. The dendritic cell has the ability to travel around to various tissues as well as the lymphatic organs. It presents the antigen on the MHC-2, and then it needs to find the cell which matches this antigen. This is going to be a B lymphocyte or a helper T lymphocyte. Of course, a lot of these are going to be hanging around the lymph nodes so the dendritic cell goes there.

Once a mate is found that B-cell or helper T cell is activated. But that is not enough. Before a B cell, which makes the antibodies, can become fully activated, it must find the T cell that also has that antigen. The T helper cell must also find its specific antigen to be activated. Once activated, the B cell begins reproducing other B cells with the same antigen Some of these turn into plasma cells which make antibodies, some into memory B cells who are going to hang around for years, and if they encounter the antigen again can skip the getting activated part and just start making antibodies. Likewise, the T cells form memory cells. Activated T cells are responsible for regulating the lymphatic system They both stimulate production and suppress production.

One other thing about the B lymphocyte. It can bind to the antigen floating around it is looking for, engulf this antigen, and present the antigen on its own MHC-2 complex. Then all it needs is to find the matching helper T cell to become fully activated. It can skip the part in which it mates with the dendritic cell and go directly to mating with the activated T cell which has the same antigen.

This seems to be a lot of trouble to go through to get these cells activated. The adaptive immune system is a powerful tool in fighting infection (and cancer). Once activated, a B lymphocyte, now called a plasma cell, can make 1000 antibody particles a second. Remember that an infected covid cell can produce up to 1 billion virions a day. You want to make sure you are making the correct antibody. (I will explain later that although the cell can make that many virions, it ends up only one in 10,00 turns into a fully infective virion. It has been calculated that plasma cells can make about 700 antibody particles per infective virion) You can see how potent the adaptive immune system can be in fighting infection. You can also see how particular it can be in that the antibody only binds to a very specific portion of the virus. If you have an antibody against a portion of the spike protein in covid which can prevent the spike protein from binding to the ACE receptor, you have enough antibody present to markedly decrease the infective ability of the spike protein.

At the same time, if the covid virus undergoes a mutation such that the spike protein only changes a few amino acids, the antibody may not bind at all to the spike and the antibody is now useless.

Your body is always being assaulted by viruses and bacteria. They have developed all kinds of mechanisms to try to overcome the defenses in your immunologic system. You win almost all the time. Most people live to be about 70. By then your lymphatic system had fought many battles and eventually won. Even with covid, 99% of the people who get infected eventually recover, at least with the current variant.

You were created to win most of the time, but you can see this is a delicate balance. A virus which gets a mutation which gives it a little advantage results in an epidemic. A little defect in your immune system may allow the pathogen to survive much longer. Evolutionary dynamics drives the bacterium or virus to reproduce as many particles as possible. You must adapt to eventually win.

This is why little adjustments on your part make a difference. Vitamin D may assist you with covid. Exercise may or may not help a little, Fasting may slightly increase autophagy. An appropriate diet may enhance your ability to generate antibodies more rapidly. These little actions or your part may swing the balance a little such that you get better faster, do not get as sick, or perhaps live instead of die. We do not have a magic bullet, but we do have common sense.

Finally, we need to review the concept of training the innate immunity system as this will play a role in Dr. Bossche's paper. Cells of the innate immune system have what are called pattern recognition receptors. These recognize molecular patterns on particles or damaged cells and respond by engulfing the particle, immobilizing the particle, killing the pathogen or cell, with the production of cytokines. Cytokine are peptides released by cells that stimulate inflammation. This attracts cells of the immune system such as neutrophils. They essentially are intracellular messengers that coordinate the innate immune response.

IgM antibodies are always around responding to the initiation of the innate response by binding to generalized antigens. Like the IgG from the adaptive system, these can immobilize antigens and cause them to clump together, enhancing removal. The IgM also has the ability to activate the complement system. And do not forget the NK (natural killer) cells of the innate system. You also have some cytotoxic T lymphocytes which can destroy abnormal cells they encounter without having been activated by specific antigens.

The NK lymphocytes recognize a range of antigens, unlike the cytotoxic lymphocytes which are much more selective, but can mount an overwhelming response which is much more sensitive to a small change in the antigen.

All of these components are enhanced the longer the foreign substance is present and IgM levels rise as the infection continues.

Recall the adaptive system which produces IgG antibodies does not really become activated against a new antigen for about three weeks. The IgM continues to rise till the IgG begins being produced. The adaptive system is quite potent as it produces a large amount of antibody (more than IgM) that is directed toward a specific antigen and will stay at a high level till the antigen is markedly diminished. We have gone over the actions of this IgG which is mainly directed to identify virions or cells presenting this antigen which activated the system, and hence enables the cells of the innate system along with activated cytotoxic T lymphocytes to destroy these particles or infected cells.

The cells of the innate system destroy particles or cells that are marked with an antibody, regardless of the antigen. This includes any antibody whether IgA, IgG, or IgM.

Another big benefit of the adaptive system is memory recall. Once the adaptive system has been activated against a specific antigen, it can rapidly be reactivated should the antigen re-appear. It retains this ability for many years, sometimes a lifetime. Should the antigen re-appear, the innate system does its usual thing but now is soon assisted by the adaptive system.

I told you not all antigens end up activating the adaptive system. The antigen must be around a while. If it is eliminated quickly, it is not worth the body's effort to go through the trouble of activating the adaptive system.

We used to think the innate system did not have this adaptive system memory , which is the basis for vaccines, but now think maybe it has something similar. Some animals do not have the adaptive system (just the innate) yet it seems their innate system has some recall. It does appear they can provide some protection against re-infection.

We have known for quite a while that giving the BCG vaccine, a vaccine from the tuberculosis bacterium, seems to activate the innate system against lipopolysaccharides, a component of many bacteria cells walls. Antibodies are not formed but a repeat exposure will stimulate the innate system to react more strongly.

In previous books I taught about epigenetics, the differential expression of DNA depending on the environment. I was talking about diet affecting epigenetics, but the innate immune systems response seems to mediate its memory through epigenetic changes in DNA expression. This is not really a memory, and the effect may only last a couple years, yet we can refer to this effect as training of the innate system.

We now have several studies showing that BCG vaccine, measles vaccine, or polio vaccine have beneficial-protective effects against infections other than the ones directed by the vaccine. In other countries children often receive the BCG vaccine, and it can be shown that this induces non-specific activation of innate immune cells. This is not adaptive immunity, and the effect only lasts a year or so.

I have used BCG as an example, and in fact there is evidence that the BCG vaccine may work as well as the covid vaccine. Not through developing antibodies, but by enhancing the innate response.

As Dr. Bossche will discuss, just raising the covid antibodies numerous times by vaccines, boosters, or repeat infections may be diminishing the beneficial effect of the adaptive immune system. Enhancing the innate system does not follow this pathway.

Different variants of covid are now relatively unaffected by a rise in original antibodies against the original strain of covid.as they do not work as well against them, but those antibodies may still be decreasing the innate response. Remember the innate response against a certain antigen is dampened in the presence of high IgG levels against that antigen. The rapid rise in IgG antibody response using the mRNA vaccine means the innate system does not have time for sufficient training.

Vaccines

Quick review. A virus enters the body. A white cell (macrophage, leukocyte, dendritic cell) engulfs this virus as it recognizes it as foreign. It digests the virus somewhat and a string of peptides are presented on the membrane of the cell. These are identified by certain T cells, and cell immunity develops in which other T cells either engulf particles expressing this antigen or destroy the cells infected with this antigen. Other cells such as dendritic cells also can engulf this antigen, process it, and present them to B cells which begins antibody formation. Antibodies are formed against very specific antigens. These attach to the epitopes, the part of the antigen to which the antibody has been sensitized, and either prevent the virus from entering the cells, prevents cell to cell spread of the virus, attach directly to the virus, or mark the cells containing these viruses to be destroyed.

The memory cells of the adaptive system enables your immune system to react quickly if you ever get this virus again. We would rather you never get sick with the virus in the first place. We could kill the virus before injecting it into you such that the immune system would recognize this virus without your having to get sick (make a vaccine), or maybe we could give you milder form or the virus which would protect you from a more severe virus.

Over the years we have gotten good at giving you protection without giving you disease. I made it sound easy, but it is quite complicated to do this and developing an acceptable vaccine takes years. Testing to make sure it works takes years. Manufacturing the vaccine also takes a while. Usually not years for certainly six months. After we make it and start giving it to people, it may take our giving a million people the vaccine to make sure there are no unanticipated side effects.

Everyone reading this will recall hearing about covid in Jan 2020. We now know that it originated in China from from a viral lab that was experimenting with this virus and attempting to develop a gain of function of the virus. There have been other books written about its origin; most agree this was a genetically modified virus.

No matter, the virus spread rapidly in the US and the deaths began accumulating. It was declared a pandemic, which is a worldwide epidemic. Now what to do?

Epidemics have existed throughout human history. A noteworthy one was the Spanish Flu 1918 – 1919. We have treated them all the same. We almost always quarantined the sick. This makes sense as even long ago we recognized contact as a factor in the spread. If there was an insect vector, we would get rid of insects. If it was related to sanitation, we fixed that. If it was bacterial, we began treatment. Over the last one hundred years or so we have advised the infected people to wear masks in public as we recognized droplet spread. If there was a vaccine, we gave everyone the vaccine.

Every time the epidemic eventually went away. By that I mean a bunch of people stopped getting sick and dying, not that the illness vanished from the earth. We figured out this was accomplished through herd immunity. Enough people, (or animals) got the illness, survived, and then did not get the illness again. If this happens to enough people, the virus is unable to spread, and it ceases to be an epidemic. We can thank the memory B cells. If activated, the IgG is generated, and your body can eliminate the virion before it produces enough virions to be able to infect someone else. A few cells may get infected, but you must have lots of infected cells in your body before you are contagious.

Like the Spanish flu, a lot of people must become infected and, although most recover, many may die before herd immunity happens. As we would expect, those who we not the healthiest were usually the ones that did not survive the illness and contribute to the herd immunity. (For the Spanish flu this amounted to about 1% of the population in the US.

Of course, if the virus is not deadly, like most influenza, only a bunch of people must catch the virus. In history, almost every time your recover from the illness causing the epidemic, you do not catch it again, hence herd immunity must eventually occur.

The Spanish influenza virus was also deadly to young healthy people in that it overactivated the immune system via a "cytokine storm". This also happens in covid, but usually to older individuals. By the way, we now have the genotype of that influenza virus and can re-create the virus. We do not know why it affected so many younger people. Let us hope we have not farmed out gain of function experiments for that virus.

In early 2020 many people were dying from covid (probably covid although not everyone was tested. It took a while to get enough tests). The treatment was the same as every epidemic, which is supportive therapy. Let's try to keep you alive till you get over the disease. There was no vaccine. The anti-viral therapy was not very good. We did quarantine the sick like we had always done. We had them wear masks. We closed the schools like we had done before. But in our modern age of medicine, we expected more, and we were not content to wait for eventual herd immunity. We expected anyone who survived covid would not get it again.

We rapidly developed a new type of vaccine, rapidly manufactured it, and rapidly distributed it throughout the country. At the time of my writing this, around 85% of adults have been vaccinated.

The vaccines were rushed through. We would not have been able to do this ten years ago, but medical science had advanced. The choice was to use a maybe not perfect vaccine or wait around for herd immunity to develop and live with the current death count. Another option was just to wait till a better vaccine was developed, but that may have taken another year.

We have heard of the mRNA vaccines. Essentially, the mRNA of the covid virus is inserted into the cell. With a real covid infection, the entire genome is inserted in the cell. The mRNA vaccines only insert a portion of the genome. Hence, we are not infecting people with the virus as this portion does not contain the entire genome and cannot make a new virus.

There are various ways to insert this piece of RNA, but the result is the same. Once inserted this piece of RNA will find its way to the ribosome and the protein coded by this piece will be produced. In a real infection the whole virus is reproduced, enveloped, and transported to the cell surface. In the RNA vaccine, the protein is made and then treated like any other antigen that is in the cell. That is the protein which contains about 1200 amino acids is broken down into peptides about 8-10 amino acids long. This is then attached to the MHC molecule we talked about last chapter and transported to the cell membrane. The T cells recognize the MHC molecule and engulfs the peptide attached to be processed by the immune system, either by sensitizing killer T cells or presenting to B cells for antibody production. Recall most cells are presenting viral antigens on the MHC-1 complex, the antigen presenting cells on the MHC-2 complex.

This is in general how the covid vaccines work. Antigens are created from mRNA. What is this mRNA coding for? The mRNA in the vaccines is coding for the spike protein which contains 1273 amino acids. In the S1 subunit we previously discussed, the part involved in binding to the ACE2 receptor, amino acids 14-685 (we number the amino acids) are the important one for my purposes. That is the binding of the virion to the receptor. The S2 subunit (686-1273) is involved with the fusion of the virion with the cell. The covid genome codes for 29 proteins. Only 4 make up the structure, but these could also be used as antigens. These are the membrane protein, the envelope, the nucleocapsid protein, and of course the spike protein The other

25 are involved in how the virus assembles copies of itself and various enzymes. We rightfully confined our attention to the spike protein as we want to prevent infection from starting or spreading. So the vaccine does not contain all the available antigens that a natural infection would.

*79If someone had covid, they would develop antibodies to the four surface proteins. If you get the mRNA vaccine, you only develop antibodies to the spike protein. Hence you can determine if you got the spike antibodies from an infection or just from the vaccine.

The Pfizer vaccine and Moderna vaccine both insert mRNA for the spike protein derived from the original Wuhan corona virus. There are slight differences in the vaccine mRNA involving start and stop signals for the ribosome, but the genotype for the spike protein is the same. As time has gone one, we have realized that the spike proteins from the mRNA vaccine is not exactly the same. What this means is that all the antibodies are not exactly the same. As we learn more about long covid, this seems to make a difference.

Johnson uses a harmless virus to transport a segment of DNA to the nucleus. This is transcribed to mRNA and sent to the ribosomes. We end up at the same place as the other vaccines. The segment transcribes for the same original spike protein. Oxford-AstraZeneca is similar but uses a different virus.

Novavax vaccine is more like classic vaccine. It is made from the spike protein itself and injected along with adjuvants to enhance stimulation of the immune system. The protein spike is the same one everyone else is using. This may stimulate the innate (cellular) immune system a little better than the others.

All of them work as advertised, that is, they stimulate the production of antibodies against the spike protein. Everyone is using the original Wuhan spike protein.

Now think back to the previous few pages. What happens when a virus enters the body? It is recognized by macrophages and dendritic cells as being foreign. It is then engulfed. The virus or protein is then processed, that is it is digested into fragments about 8-12 amino acids long. These fragments are presented to the surface of the cell attached to MHC molecules (MHC 1 or MHC 2) which T cells recognize, take up the attached antigen, and eventually end up with antibodies or activated killer lymphocytes against these antigens.

So, when I say you make antibodies against covid, you do not make one antibody against the entire spike protein, but rather lots of different antibodies against the antigens in that protein. Even if we are only interested in the S1 subunit of the spike protein, that's still about 700 amino acids. You can see we can end up with a lot of different antigens and hence antibodies.

We can test to see if these vaccines work by taking plasma from someone who has received a vaccine and see if that plasma which contains all the antibodies inhibits the virus. We can also compare that plasma with the plasma of someone who has recovered from a natural covid infection and never had the vaccine.

We don't really have to know which specific antibody; just does it work or not. Now we could find out the details if we want, but that is for developing monoclonal antibody therapy.

It ends up your adaptive immune system is exquisitely selective with these antigens. You can have two antigens that differ in only one amino acid and the antibody will bind to one but not the other. You can also have a deletion in the antigen, which is missing an amino acid, and that may affect the binding. You could also have an antibody to a peptide of a few amino acids, and that peptide may coincidentally be found in another protein and the antibody may bind to that, even though it has nothing to do with covid.

The vaccines worked great (initially). There were few major side effects in adults. It caused almost everyone to substantially increase anti covid antibodies. They appeared to not only protect you from infection, but also decrease the severity of an infection They worked exactly as we thought they would. We expected them to work like any historical vaccine, that is it would keep you from getting infected and hence spreading the virus which would result in herd immunity without having a bunch of people die to get that herd immunity. Why am I writing this book?

We know RNA viruses get more mutations. The cell is quite good at accurately using transcription to convert the DNA code into RNA. It is not quite as good following the mRNA message. All the covid vaccines have developed antibodies against antigens found in the original covid virus, SARS CoV-2 Wuhan. You can imagine that if some mutations have occurred in the spike protein that has infected you, that these antibodies may not work as well. When I say mutations, that usually means one of the amino acids has been replaced by another, or that one of the amino acids has been deleted, or maybe some amino acids have been added. That may be all it takes to make the neutralizing antibody, which is the antibody that keeps the virus from infecting us, from working as well, as the antibody may not attach or block that antigen, which due to a mutation is not exactly the same as the original spike protein, as well and prevent the receptor from binding to the spike protein.

The mutation may be one that makes it easier to bind to the receptor or makes it easier for the virion to enter the cell, or maybe makes it more efficient in making more virions. If a mutation makes the virion more efficient, it will eventually become the dominant genome. If it makes it more infectious, it will become the main type of genome, that is variant, in the community.

Before we go on, let me define the efficacy and effectiveness of a vaccine. If you have a clinical trial and you are comparing the vaccinated people verses the unvaccinated, that is got a placebo (double blind trial) , you don't care about how many in total got infected, but rather you want to compare how many vaccinated got the disease vs. how many of the placebo go the disease.

If you have a thousand people in the study and 50 in the vaccinated group got covid but 100 in the placebo group, that means you reduced the chance of getting infected with vaccination by 50%. Thus, you had an efficacy of 50%. Effectiveness is not the same as efficacy. It is how well the vaccine works in real life, not in a clinical study.

For a vaccine to get approved, they must have an efficacy of at least 50%. The efficacy does not tell us how many people got covid, it just tells us how well it works vs placebo. Effectiveness may be lower in the real world because you will be giving the vaccine to people who may be older and sicker than in a clinical trial.

All the vaccines started out with an efficacy of around 90%, and an effectiveness not far behind. As we all know, right now that is not true. Some have now dropped below 50% with the emergence of new variants.

Now let me explain the naming of the variants.

When SARS CoV-2 came on the scene, genotyping was performed. Just a few years ago genotyping, that is determining the nucleoside composition of a viral gene, was not an easy task and took a bit of time. Now laboratories all over the world genotype viruses. WHO noted many different genotypes pouring in as numerous different ones were constantly developing. We decided just to pay particular attention to variants of concern. That is new genotypes that may lead to increased infections. Here is a brief record.

Original or wild type or natural

Alpha (B.1.1.7 lineage)

Beta (B.1.351)

Delta (B.1.617.2)

Omicron (B1.1.529, BA.1, BA.2, BA.3, BA.4, BA.5)

Each letter is more infective or deadly than the previous version. (There are others, but I am paying attention to those in the USA)

These are the variants that have caused surges in cases or deaths in the US. There are many variants but in general we are only interested in the ones that are more infective or deadly. Mutations cause increased virulence and infectivity, and these are just the most prominent amount many versions of the virus. We can get the genotype of the viruses and know where the mutations are located. We can now predict the behavior of the virus just on that knowledge.

Alpha: 8 mutations on spike protein subunit 1

Beta 9 mutations

Delta 8 mutations

Omicron 50 mutations, 26 unique to this variant

These mutations may be cumulative.

Each of these mutations moved the spike protein further away from the original genotype to which the vaccine antibodies are directed. Each of these variants was more infective than the original. It was easily noted that the neutralizing antibodies developed by the vaccine did not work nearly as well. You took plasma from a vaccinated person, exposed it to the variant, and it did not respond to the antibodies, which are the neutralizing antibodies Those that inhibited infection. Sometimes falling below 50% effectiveness.

Over the last year many new variants have developed such that I no longer keep track of them. You might ask why we do not just produce a new vaccine every time a new variant occurs. The reason is that they are changing so rapidly that by the time a new one is developed to the point where they have been manufactured in bulk, that variant is no longer dominant. A new booster is to be issued next month. It already has fallen to less than 10% of the infections, and by next month will be close to 1%

The effectiveness of the neutralizing antibodies is not an absolute event. A higher level of these antibodies works a little better by competing for the antibody sites on the spike proteins. As these antigenic sites change, the old antibodies did not bind as well. Sometimes not at all. There were new mutations that changed the antigen, and the vaccine did not generate new antibodies to these new sites. You are stuck with the antibodies the vaccine produced.

If you got a natural infection, and had not been previously vaccinated, you produced somewhat different antibodies as the variants took over the infections. We have gone through several rounds of infections, and now the variants do not cross react with each other. The antigens and antibodies are different. If you get one type of variant, it may not protect you fully from another type.

That is not to say the original antibodies are useless. Although the neutralizing antibody levels and their effectiveness decline with time, additional shots, that is boosters, or exposure to infection will increase the levels. Higher levels correlate with slightly more protection, but overall, as time goes on and the variants emerge, breakthrough infections or re-infections become likely. This is especially true with the omicron variant. Now we estimate a booster will give you about one to two months protection from getting covid till the not extremely effective antibody drops to a low enough level that it no longer protects you. An effective antibody would mean that the antibody level would have to drop much lower to lose protection, and hence last much longer.

Right now, there is discussion as to whether the boosters should add antigens appropriate to the B.4 and B.5 omicron variants. That is to add another different mRNA to the original. By the time the booster comes out, these variants may be long gone. We can make the mRNA boosters and vaccines faster, but it still takes a few months to get the in the supply system. On Nov 5, 2022, Omicron BA.5 was about 65% of the variants. Two months previously it was 95%. Of course now it is zero.

We have long known that if you have adaptive memory against a particular antigen, exposure to a similar antigen will stimulate a response, meaning it will begin making antibodies. It will also prevent the development of new, different antibodies unless the new antigen is significantly different from the memory antigen. You get old antibodies for new antigens and may not make any new antibodies against the variants.

In other words if your adaptive system has already created antibodies to specific antigens, it will not go through the trouble of making brand new antibodies against that antigen unless the antigen is substantially different. The spike protein has over 1200 amino acids, and lots of antigens. Most of these have not changed, and hence the antibodies that were developed are the same as the original. Evolutionary dynamics does not drive mutations to succeed unless that mutation creates a specific advantage to spread the virus. Hence a mutation that does not involve the spike protein such that it increases that mutation to become dominant, will not become incorporated in the new genome. Hence most of the time your body is not making new different antibodies.

We have people vaccinated with antibodies against the original virus and initially those antibodies seemed to work fine. As additional variants came along, the old antibodies did not prevent infection, yet these new antigens were close enough that your immune system simply activated memory cells instead of creating new, different antibodies. We now have people who have been infected with several different variants yet did not develop antibodies against these variants.

This is not an absolute process. If the antigen level of a new variant goes high enough, your body may make some new antibodies. But even these do not tend to respond as well if you already have the old antibodies around. The old antibiotics may interfere with bonding of new antibiotics.

You have someone who just got over Omicron BA.5. We now know they only get 1-2 months of protection. That infection boosted their antibody levels to the original stalk protein. Maybe it generated a few new antibodies to the Omicron stalk protein, but maybe not.

Say we add the Omicron BA.5 stalk antigens to the vaccine. We know the mRNA vaccines seem to generate the production of stalk antigens such that more are present than if you got the natural infection and had never gotten the vaccine. We are hoping this high level of antigens will provoke some new antibodies more specific to Omicron BA.5.

Of course, we do not know if the Omicron BA.5 variant will be the most prominent variant by the time this vaccine is released.

There is also a risk involved in adding BA.5 antigens that I have not heard anyone mentioning. We know the original vaccine seemed to work fine initially. But it did not work well enough to sterilize the virus. That is, it took a while to eliminate the virus from the body. Immune pressure means the antibodies are working well enough to eliminate some of the virus, but ongoing mutations of the virus as they are being generated continues to select spike proteins generated through mutations that will survive the antibodies. These mutated stalk proteins that are part of the new virions, will eventually become prominent as the older virions are ceasing to exist because the antibodies are affecting them. You can see how this drives a higher population of these mutant virions since they are the ones surviving.

We get new variants resistant to the old antibodies. Evolutionary dynamics is also driving higher infectiousness. The longer the virus is allowed to reproduce in the body, the more likely a new variant will develop. The more infectiousness, the more virus particles are being produced which also increases the chances of new variants.

If you add BA.4 and BA.5 stalk proteins to the original vaccine, you may induce a few more antibodies against Omicron. It is highly unlikely these will be sterilizing antibodies. Now you have highly infectious Omicron, antibodies that may work a little, but still have many people catching covid. You are creating immune pressure to get a better variant to develop. When you get a new variant, they are almost always more infectious as they must outcompete the old variant. This is easier if you are handicapping the old variant with new antibodies that work a little.

You will get new variants. They probably will be more infectious. The vaccines will not work. Currently a covid infection is mild. This is related to the genotype of the virus and the interaction of the antibodies with dendritic cells to inhibit systemic infection. It is said the vaccine is working because it is keeping the infection mild. Of course, this same vaccine did not keep the Delta variant mild.

Omicron became dominant not because the disease was milder, but because the infectiousness was higher. The vaccine induced antibody dependent enhancement of infection. It so happened that this also reduced virulence. Dr Bossche will explain that these two characteristics of the virus do not have to exist together.

There is always a temptation to anthropomorphize, that is give human characteristics to the virus. Evolutionary dynamics of all living things is driven by the principle to produce more of that living thing. Some may say this is the reason Omicron is milder because if people only get sick but do not die, this allows more viruses to exist and thus satisfies the evolutionary drive, especially since they can get re-infected. The virus would never become highly virulent because then it would kill more people and hence spread less. The virus would have to be crazy to start killing everyone.

Viruses do not think. They do not try to figure things out. They are not sane and do not go crazy. The winner of virus evolution is the one that produces more virions. A more virulent variant may produce more virions in an individual. You may say I am crazy to say that because it would be viral suicide if it killed everyone.

That has never happened in recorded history. Currently in the US, the virus has killed about a third of one percent of the population. It has affected us, but mainly through government actions, not because there were not enough people to keep the economy running. Less than 1% of the population of the US died as a result of the Spanish Flu.

If a variant developed that was twenty times as lethal as Omicron, it would still not disrupt the fabric of society. If we examine the black plague, a bacterial instead of a viral infection, which occurred about 700 years ago, it appears somewhere between 10-30% of the people must die before society deteriorates. This is primarily because there is not enough food produced. In recorded history, famine appears to be the major cause of death.

There has been much discussion as to how many people needed to get the vaccine to develop herd immunity. At that time, it was not well known that the vaccine was not providing immunity to the people getting it. We estimated about 30 to 50% of people needed to be vaccinated, assuming that vaccination prevented getting covid. Or that many get the disease, if getting covid prevented you from getting it again, to achieve herd immunity. If neither of these were true, would it take 30-50% of the people dying to get herd immunity? ****

This started out with our thinking the vaccine would work great. For some reason it did not and began mutating at a high rate. Something we did not expect. New variants came about every few months to which the vaccine was progressively less effective. This is not something we had seen before. The vaccine also never provided sterilization, which is once you got covid you did not get it again. Also, once you got the vaccine, you still got covid.

It is now believed that the Wuhan virus escaped from the viral laboratory. The US was probably funding gain of function of this virus. The laboratory succeeded and developed a virus which was more infective in humans and had additional amino acids at the furin cleavage site. The changes made may have increased the propensity for mutation, hence the observed rapid development of new variants. The genetic changes may also have inhibited sterilization antibodies from developing which again increased the mutation rate, by allowing the virus to linger longer in humans.

Even if this is all true, it does not make any difference now, but I think we should include these assumptions in our development of future treatment plans.

Do not forget the reason I am writing this book. I am trying to teach you enough of the language so that you can understand the paper by Dr. Bossche. It is not that I may agree with everything he says, or that the paper is going to change vaccine science, but rather it has seemed to me that there have been no other voices that have been heard that are in disagreement with what the government and FDA have been advocating. It's almost like these voices have been intentionally silenced.

It appears the main reason these views may have been silenced is that the paper is against the policy of mass and mandated vaccination. He believes this is making the epidemic worse, and in fact, most would agree that we are no closer to herd immunity now than we were in Jan 2020.

The paper is not easily understood unless you are heavily involved in the field, which means this is about .0001% of the adults between 18 and 75. I think I can get most of you up to the point where you will understand what he is talking about and how he arrived at his conclusions. Even if you do not agree, it will help you understand the language of covid and be able to decide for yourself what you should be doing.

Let me add I am not reproducing the paper in this book. I will give you his conclusions. You can easily find a PDF of the paper online. I do have another book, *Covid and Vaccines for Medical Professionals*, if you want to read the paper with my commentary throughout to help even medical professionals to understand. Of course, if you are a virologist, just read the original paper.

GLYCOSYLATION

A few of you have read some of my books in which I mention AGEs, which is advanced glycated end products. This is a process in which glucose, fructose, or some other sugar is attached to a protein or fat in a non-enzymatic manner. The poster boy for this process is the hemoglobin A1c molecules.

In this molecule a sugar, usually glucose, is attached to the hemoglobin molecule. No enzyme is used. Once attached, it stays there. We do not have the enzyme to separate it. It ends up the amount of attachment is related to the glucose level. The red blood cells usually last about 3 months so we can calculate the average glucose level in the blood over the last three months by measuring the A1c.

AGES accumulate in your body. They are related to the amount of glucose in the blood. Since we usually do not have the enzyme that attaches the sugar, and it can be attached to various locations throughout a large molecule, it is difficult to digest the molecule. These glycated molecules can cause problems throughout the body like stiffening of the blood vessels and skin or inducing inflammation.

Your body can use various proteolytic enzymes to try to chop them up into smaller pieces, and sometimes you can get rid of them in the urine. There is also the process of autophagy that occurs in almost all cells which allows the cell to identify the ages and digest them for energy or building blocks.

The process that forms AGEs is **glycation**. We are going to talk about **glycosylation**, which is the attachment of a linear or branched monosaccharides, usually not glucose, to another molecule through an enzyme. Your body does this on purpose. Glycation and Glycosylation may be involved in the poor prognosis of those with diabetes and covid. The higher the glucose level, the more of both of these processes you get. Increases of both or either my change the conformation of proteins enough that it encourages trans infection enabling the virus to enter the cell membrane under conditions of low amounts of ACE2 receptors which exist in the lower respiratory tract as well as other distant sites. This is associated with severe disease.

A glycan is a bunch of monosaccharides linked together in the endoplasmic reticulum of the cell. You normally make these. In N-linked glycosylation, these are then attached to an asparagine amino acid on a protein. There is also an O-linked glycosylation which uses the amino acid serine, , or threonine as the attachment. There can be many different glycans attached to a protein. The cells in your body normally have glycans attached to their membranes.

The virions also have some glycans attached to their membranes. Glycans are often used by your body to identify your cells. Viruses have adapted this and may use different glycans to try to hide from the immune system.

These glycans are manufactured in your body. Unlike AGEs, they do not appear spontaneously. Glycoprotein is a protein attached to glycan.

These glycoproteins serve many purposes, often as an identifier to which other cell receptors attach. This is used by the immune system to determine if the cell is foreign and needs to be destroyed. The glycoproteins assist molecules in conforming to their correct structure. Proteins come in many shapes and often may be folded. In order for an enzyme to attach to a protein, it must fit into the proper slot. Glycoproteins can change the topography of the protein to either encourage or discourage actions of enzymes.

For our purposes the virion has glycoproteins attached to keep the body from recognizing it as an invader. If we look at the covid spike protein, it has glycoproteins attached, both to hide from antibodies or promote a better configuration to attach to the cells receptor.

Remember the virus relies on the cell to make proteins and glycans . Each cell type may make slightly different glycans. These are then going to attach themselves to different parts of the spike protein which may obstruct antibody attachment, or in some cases encourage receptor attachment and subsequent engulfing of the virus into the cell.(endocytosis).

The glycans attached to the virus were made by the cell. Hence, they are identified as the cell and may then mask an immune response.

I don't believe I am giving you a good picture. Glycoproteins can have hundreds of different compositions and thousands of different structures. An N-glycoprotein occurring at identical sites on a different spike protein may have different properties due to the structure of the glycans.

Imagine the spike protein. Now think about the end that attaches to the cell receptor. Now remember there are about 600 amino acids making up this end. Now imagine attaching fuzzy tennis balls up and down this structure. You can see if we place the tennis balls in the right location, if may hide or get in the way of the antigen that an antibody is seeking. If we put some in just the right place, we may be able to hold open the leaf petal on the receptor binding portion of the stalk protein and allow it to attach to the ACE receptor easier.

We read about glycosylation in the Bossche paper. We know that evolutionary pressure continues to seek changes in the virus that will aid the purpose of the virus, which is to survive and thrive. If a mutation makes the virus more infectious, eventually that will become the most common variant.

The same is true for glycosylation. Attaching a glycan to a certain amino acid (N-glycosylation or O-glycosylation, may make it more difficult for an antibody to attach. It may change the configuration of the protein such that infection happens easier. It may even allow the virus to become more virulent.

This is a dynamic process as new mutations continually arise which allow different configurations as different glycans can be attached. O-glycosylation attaches to two different amino acids, serine or threonine. As mutations occur, some of these will switch an amino acid to one in which O-glycosylation can occur. It is the whole configuration of the virus that determines if this new arrangement is beneficial or not. Most of the time it's not, but you get a billion attempts. every day.

Innate Immunity

This is the most important part of your immune system. The cells in your body are under almost continuous attack by microbes, both bacteria and viruses; yet you do not get sick that often. Physical barriers, which is the skin, and mucous membranes, separate you from the outside. The upper respiratory tract, the lungs, and the gut is lined with cells, some of which secrete mucous. The gut is loaded with immune cells.

Most of the time this keeps the foreign antigens out. If some do penetrate, the rest of the innate immune system is activated. This is composed of cells, antibodies, various chemicals, and the compliment system.

These cells are those we are familiar with, mainly the white blood cells. These have receptors that recognize things that aren't you and take action. The neutrophils mainly engulf particles they don't recognize. At the same time, they secrete cytokines, which are chemicals, which attract other white cells, increase blood flow, and make it easier for the cells to leave the blood vessels and enter the tissue. The basophils, eosinophils neutrophils contain different chemicals. We also have the NK (natural killer) cells which identify other cells that do not look right. It then kills the cells by secreting enzymes and chemicals which induce the cells to undergo apoptosis (cell death). These cells engulf bacteria and parts of other cells.

Your body is very efficient doing this. Most of the time the adaptive immune system does not get involved. You do not start making antibodies against antigens unless they linger around awhile. If we start infecting you with a virus today, the IgG antibodies which are specific to that antigen will not appear for about 3 weeks. They then appear in large quantities, and you develop memory cells so that if you see that antigen again, you do not have to wait 3 weeks.

In the meantime, your innate system is getting rid of the antigens so that most of the time these antibodies never even need to develop.

The adaptive immune system is a powerful tool in that it can flood the body with specific antibodies. The purpose of these antibodies is to attach to abnormal antigens. The antibody itself does not kill any virion or infected cell, it does identify this particle so that your innate immune system can engulf them, destroy the cells, or activate the compliment system to destroy them. There is such a level of antibodies that practically all these antigens will be identified and marked. The memory aspect of the adaptive system means that within a few days these antibodies will be present.

The innate system does have a memory aspect. The IgM produced reacts to a broad range of antigens, not the specific ones that the adaptive reacts to. Still, it can get some specification such as being sensitized to lipopolysaccharides which may be present in several different antigens. The B1a lymphocytes make the IgM antibody, and these lymphocytes can increase the amount of those IgM antibodies that are produced upon exposure to certain antigens. It can also increase the cytotoxic lymphocytes specificity to these antigens. The memory does not last a lifetime like the adaptive system, but it does seem to last a few years.

Let me review a couple topics that are mentioned in the paper. Dr. Bossche mentions "training" the innate immune system. No matter what, you depend on the innate system to destroy the virus and virus infected cells. The adaptive system identifies these antigens which make them much easier to get rid of. The adaptive system antibodies can also bind to portions of the virus such that they cannon bind and enter the cell, thus cells do not get infected to start with.

If the antibodies become unable to bind to their specific antigens, they may not be preventing infection, and may actually be enhancing infection. Without a well-functioning innate system, you will have difficulty clearing the virus, and hence the infection lasts longer.

When you initially get infected, the IgM begins binding to cells and viruses. As I said before, this is not as specific as the adaptive system. After about three weeks the adaptive system begins to generate IgG antibodies. This signals the innate system to cut back on IgM. By then, the innate system has already begun to enhance production of those IgMs that have been attracted to the infecting virus. The IgG suppresses the production of IgM, because if everything is going right, it is no longer needed for this virus.

If this is a reinfection with the same virus, the IgG memory goes into action and within a few days you get lots of specific IgG. This then tends to suppress IgM production The IgM to this virus has been hanging around. The IgG fell to a low level once the antigen was eliminated but will rapidly boost production should the antigen re-appear and the IgM, which never went away, is unable to eliminate the antigen.

The less specific to a particular antigen IgM was boosted as a result of the initial infection. Unlike the specific IgG, this elevated IgM can bind to other viruses or antigens that may not be the same initial virus, but close enough that it will work. So that if you had a covid variant , the IgM will be able to attach to this variant. If you had IgG to the original covid virus, that IgG may not be able to be effective against the variant.

If you are vaccinated and you get a covid variant whose spike protein is different from the original spike protein, your nonspecific IgM will still be useful in the destruction of the virus since the antigen does not have to be specific like is does with the IgG.

You make plenty of IgG which will tend to suppress the IgM which is the antibody doing all the work. Most people who get covid will survive, but it takes longer to clear the virus than if they had effective

IgG. Of course, this may encourage more mutations as the viruses are around longer, and it possibly predispose you to "long" covid.

You will not make much of a brand-new IgG with infection of a variant which happens to poorly bind that old spike protein. The antigens are similar enough that your body will revive the old memory cells to make the old antibody.

In the innate system, a new variant will stimulate production of the previous IgM, but since this IgM is not highly specific like IgG, it will function against the new variant, despite all the non-working neutralizing IgG antibody around.

It does take exposure to the antigen for a while to educate the innate system. If you get a natural infection, and have not had the vaccine, by the time the IgG memory cells are produced the antigen has been around long enough that the innate system is educated.

If your innate system worked so well that the antigen disappeared in a short period of time, you would never have the necessity for IgG production.

If you were vaccinated, you had elevated levels of the spike protein antigens, and your body rapidly triggered IgG production such that the innate system was never trained against the original covid antigens, your innate system will be hindered against any re-infection. Eventually Dr. Bossche believes the vaccine will become useless, and those who were vaccinated will be at increased risk, not only for re-infection but for severe disease. You will not get immunity to covid. It you were not vaccinated; you have preserved your innate system memory and ability to possibly reach a sterilization immunity.

This is partly from education of the innate system, and partly because you will not be promoting a burst of IgG antibodies every time you get a booster, get re-infected, or even exposed to the virus. The elevated levels of ineffective neutralizing antibodies may interfere with the action of the non-specific IgM antibodies which are effective and thus the IgG may be hindering the IgM from binding to the spike protein. In other words the IgG which does not work well and is at a high level will interfere with the IgM which does work well The IgG levels when boosted are much higher than the IgM levels.

The dendritic cell is a part of the innate system. Its job is to engulf antigens and present these antigens on MHC to the lymph nodes to activate cells there. This cell travels through the lymph system to various lymphatic areas to achieve this function.

Dr. Bossche believes this is a major source of covid infection to organs outside the upper respiratory tract. This cell can bind whole virions to its surface. Recall the MHC complexes present antigens to other cells. These antigens are pieces of the virion. Whole virions, not just the antigens pieces, can infect cells in the usual ways. Thus antigens cannot infect cells.

These whole, infective virions can become attached to the dendritic cell membrane and are free to leave and infect other cells. Since the dendritic cell travels in the body, it can spread this infective virions.

The upper respiratory tract cells are exposed to free virions that have entered the mucous membrane and start bouncing off the cells looking for receptors. As we get to the lower respiratory tract, there are not very many free virions, hence not as many cells get infected.

Virions on the dendritic cell may be the main transport mechanism for covid viruses.to encourage systemic infection. It does not appear that viremia is the main method by which these virions travel.

As will be explained, once a cell is infected, its neighbor can then become directly infected without needing to activate a receptor.

If you look at the mustard seed(the virus) on the basketball (the dendritic cell), , you can see how a thousand virions may be carried on one dendritic cell.

Let me go over what Dr. Bossche terms training of the innate immune system. The adaptive system creates memory cells for specific antigens. These are from both the bursa cells (B lymphocytes) which turn into plasma cells and make antibodies, and memory cells for the cytotoxic T cells specific for that antigen which destroy certain cells displaying that antigens.

The innate system does not have these memory cells. But it does have a memory. B1a cells, which make IgM, can become activated without the help of other T cells. But they can only be activated by certain general antigens such as polysaccharides, glycolipids, or nucleic acids. Most antigens are proteins which require the normal B and T cell activation. process.

The B1a cells produce IgM . When these antigens are present, IgM production ramps up. The IgM antibodies are not as specific as the IgG antibodies, but it appears certain types of IgM is produced in response to certain groups of antigens. The NK cells also seem to increase activity against certain antigens with chronic exposure. The non-specific NK cells can eliminate some of the new variants which have a mutated spike protein that is resistant to the antibodies created from the original covid spike protein, as well as and the antibodies stimulated by the mRNA covid vaccine.

Usually, the innate system B1a cells have a few weeks to be exposed to an antigen before elevated levels of IgG suppress the production of IgM. If the IgG levels rise too rapidly, such as during mass vaccination of the mRNA vaccine, the B1a cells may not receive enough exposure to the antigen to get trained. This particularly happens if you get vaccinated soon after getting or recovering from a covid infection. That is why generally we do not advise giving vaccines during the middle of an epidemic.

In general, exposure of the innate system to a specific disease in which the antigen is present for several weeks seems to enhance the immune response to that disease later. It is not a vaccination as no memory B cells are involved, but more likely is related to epigenetic changes in the B1a cells and NK cells.

Let me clarify this idea of innate immune system memory. B1a cells can be directly activated by certain antigens. These antigens appear to be those that have repeating amino acids. When these B1a cells are activated, they will produce more specific IgM antibodies. These antibodies are more specific than the regular IgM antibodies, but not as specific as the IgG antibodies. The IgM antibodies have a different shape than IgG and are larger. They also can activate the compliment system.

The B1a cells do not form memory B cells which, once activated, roam around for years looking for the antigen so that they can then start reproducing. Unlike memory cells, once the B1a cells begin producing more specific IgM, epigenetic changes in the expression of the DNA which enabled the new IgM to be produced lingers for a few years, just like it may linger in all epigenetic changes in your body. It is not permanent like a vaccine. Epigenetic changes in DNA is driven by the environment of the cell.

I mention BCG as an example of training the innate system. We know this is not permanent but does last a few years. It seems to sensitize the IgM to a general class of lipopolysaccharide.

WHY

I started writing about Diet and Health a few years ago. It started with the observation that there were lots of people with type 2 diabetes. It turns out that this is related to obesity. In fact, over 40% of the adults in the US had obesity, prediabetes, or type 2 diabetes. That seemed to be a high number.

When I examined history, it was not always like this. Whatever was causing this seemed to have appeared in the last couple hundred years. Eventually, I determined it was not a lack of exercise or an excess of food in the world, it was the diet.

The modern Western diet has induced obesity in every modern country who has adopted this diet. This led me to write numerous books and my having to teach people about diabetes, eating, fasting, metabolism, and of course diet. I then realized I had to start in the womb, which has led to books about epigenetics in pregnancy.

The point is that this started with an accepted observation, but I wanted to know why this was the case.

Now I have the chart below, that is deaths from covid since Jan 2020. I am living through this history. I remember when there was not a vaccine. Early in 2020 there was a peak of infections in New York City in which the hospitals were jammed. People were dying in the hallways and emergency rooms. There was no treatment except supportive care and ventilators, and that did not work well at all. Basically no one knew what was happening or what was going to happen.

We reverted to the historical treatment for epidemics which was to quarantine the sick. For some reason we thought masking everyone would protect us despite our only masking sick people in previous epidemics. Of course, it was soon evident that the old and immune compromised were at a much-increased risk, the same as it had been in all epidemics. Even though we also soon discovered children did not appear to be at high risk, we closed the schools. This was something we had also done in past epidemics when children were at risk. This was not the case with covid and now it appears closing the schools caused numerous problems and it was not worth the small covid benefit from the closing.

We had no vaccine, no medications, no real treatment, and a severe respiratory virus that we had not seen before. It was starting to sound like the Spanish Flu of 1918 all over again. The only way we got over that one was to wait for herd immunity at the cost of numerous lives.

You remember the business shutdown for two weeks to flatten the curve. Of course, that turned into months. I believe that was the plan all along, but no one would have agreed to do that if they had known. Now I wonder if that worked or was even a good idea, but I agreed at the time with that approach. Now I do not think that was a good idea, but hindsight is 20/20.

People were wearing masks, segregating, and staying at home; Some voluntary, some mandated. Various treatments were being tried with slight success. We were waiting for a new vaccine which was supposed to offer some hope.

The vaccine was approved in Dec 2020. This was right around the peak in the daily number of covid deaths in the US. See chart. People were standing in line to get one. We were smart enough to prioritize the elderly as they were obviously at increased risk. Another vaccine was approved in Jan 2021. The supply chain was functioning and now the CDC is on TV telling us to get the vaccine in order to stop the spread of covid and thus get us to develop herd immunity. Of course, most people were already trying to get a vaccine.

Just as we all should have been rejoicing that we had a handle on the epidemic and life would return to normal, it takes a bad turn.

The government, both state and federal, begins demanding you must get the vaccine, something we had not done before. Why would we have to do that? You would have to be crazy not to get the vaccine, or maybe not.

Every adult in the US knew what a vaccine was from personal experience. We got tetanus vaccines, we got MMR, if you were old enough you had gotten a smallpox vaccine. Many had gotten flu vaccines. We thought if you got a vaccine, it protected you from getting the disease. Sure, we knew it wasn't perfect, but it seemed worth it.

Now we had a new type of vaccine, and it was not crazy to expect it would work like any other vaccine. The CDC was telling us this every day. I and many other physicians were a little concerned in that we knew that a normal vaccine takes years to get approved. We knew that it would take a million people getting the vaccine and watching them for a year to be sure it was safe and that it worked. And this was no normal vaccine. We really had no experience with it.

But this was an emergency and it got emergency authorization for temporary approval. We knew there was a slight risk, but for the most part, for most people, the risk was probably worth the benefit. Nobody really complained too much.

Then it became mandated. That bothered some people. By now I know that if I am in good health, my risk of dying from covid is pretty low. At the same time, I don't want to get sick or have to go to the hospital, so it is probably worth it. But to make me get the vaccine whether I want it or not, well that just doesn't sound right.

The CDC on TV every day told me I had to get it otherwise grandma could catch it from you and die. I don't want grandma to die, but she got the vaccine two months ago. Why then do I have to get the vaccine to keep her from dying?

Suddenly I am starting to wonder if this new vaccine is really a vaccine. It is starting to sound a lot more like the gamma globulin shot we used to give years ago. It would keep you from getting sick for a while, and help you if you were sick, but it was no vaccine.

Now it is July 10, 2021. The new vaccine has been out about six months. I am looking at the graph the CDC puts out every week and I see cases and deaths from covid are at the lowest level they have been for over a year. The vaccine appears to be working. I may not like it, but I can't argue with success. I may not like being forced to get the shot, but I plan to go along.

A year later I looked at the chart. I did not understand what was going on. I still can remember how everyone getting forced to get the vaccine was going to be worth it. Is the current graph what all the experts predicted? I was expecting the epidemic to die out. This did not happen.

I remember the time when I was wondering why everyone is getting fat and getting diabetes. I eventually figured that out and what to do about it. Many people were doing the same thing and there are thousands of diet books. Now where are all the people explaining to me why the chart looks like this and what to do about it? Can you tell me what the chart is going to look like six months from now?

When I think back over the last year or so, I remembered that I did not read much about people questioning the effectiveness of the vaccine. Certainly not any debate. I know now there actually were people, it's just those opinions were being suppressed.; by the print media, the social media, the television media, and the state and federal governments. Physicians were being disciplined for spreading false information. Websites were shut down, People were taken off Facebook, contrary opinions were either not published anywhere or ridiculed, maybe denounced as unpatriotic. I know there were physicians that did not agree with mandating vaccines, but you could not find them.

The government and CDC still appear on TV occasionally. Everyone knows that the new vaccine is not exactly like the old vaccines. We have redefined what we mean by the vaccine working several times. The problem was blamed on those damned people who just won't get vaccinated. We estimate that around 90% of the adults in the US have been either vaccinated or have had covid. It may be more than that. If we could just get those other ones to get vaccinated this epidemic would be over

Wait a minute, the problem is those kids who have not gotten vaccinated. We may have to mandate they get the vaccine before they come to school.

Now that I think about it, the problem is those damn newborns and babies who have not been vaccinated. If we could just force everyone who has been born in the last 70 years, including those born yesterday, to get vaccinated, we would be over this epidemic.

Without a vaccine or antiviral medications, it took about two years to get herd immunity for the Spanish Flu 1918-1920. We are now approaching 3 ½ years with covid with no sign of herd immunity.

Dr. Bossche has written a paper trying to answer the question as to why the new vaccines have not solved the covid problem. The paper is difficult to read and therefore few are going to read it.

It is 45 pages of single-spaced typing. It has a poor title if you were trying to get any common person to read it. It is not in the format of a research paper with an introduction, background , methods, results, and discussion. It is not a research paper, more like an essay.

He has sprinkled 140 references throughout the book, usually following a sentence to justify a statement he has just made.

It is difficult to read in the sense it must be read carefully, and many judgments must be made by the reader as to if the statements are making any sense.

I anticipate less than one hundred people in the world are going to read the complete paper. Probably none of these are going to be outside the field of vaccines or virology.

Many more may read the title, skim through the paper, and read the summary. Probably none of these will be the audience of most of my books, the common man.

There have been a few articles about this paper. All have been dismissive and condescending. Most are written by reporters who did not read the paper except the title and summary, but did speak to an expert, who I can tell did not read the entire paper either.

I have read the paper numerous times. It takes me awhile to get through it as I must look up many things I didn't understand, never learned, forgot about, or to get a definition. I am not an expert in this field, but I will probably be the only one to actually look up all the references. I say look up but on my pdf copy on my computer, I just click on the reference.

I am not an expert. Despite the media dismissing his ideas, everyone who looks at his resume would consider Dr Bossche to be one. He is not an academic and does not work in an ivory tower. He actually has worked at real jobs.

Although I am a retired physician and have not personally examined him, he is not a wacko. He does a terrible job presenting his ideas to the common man. In all my books I believe the common man using common sense can understand most of these concepts if I just teach him the language of the subject.

I want to answer the question; why does the covid cases, hospitalizations, and death charts look like they do? What does that mean, and what can we expect?

I have written a book, *Covid and Vaccines for Medical Professionals*, in which I reproduce the paper and have given you the link to look it up yourself. If you want to get the references, you will have to get the pdf of the paper. I go through the paper line by line. I look up every reference. I often must add my own explanatory comments and add paragraphs of my own explanatory notes. . I may have clarified it for a few more people who had a solid understanding of the subject. I am talking about graduates in biological science. I think I may have succeeded in explaining it to most physicians.

The paper was designed to be read by vaccine professionals. My previous book is designed to be read by medical type professionals.

This book is written to the common man, and I do not reproduce the paper but rather explain some of the conclusions of the paper. Again, these are Dr. Bossche's conclusions.

If you have gotten to this page, I have instructed you in some basic concepts which will allow you to understand the language of the covid vaccines. You will now be able to evaluate the information you hear on TV and use your common sense.

I will give you the conclusions of the paper and predictions by Dr. Bossche.

At the end I will give my beliefs and non-expert commentary and advice. You have heard a lot in the last few years about covid vaccines, and what you should be doing. It is possible you are like me and some of the information turned out to not make any sense. Dr. Bossche's paper is just a vehicle by which I can explain what is going on and am counting on your common sense to do what is best for you.

Deaths and Cases Charts

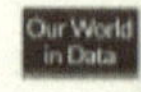

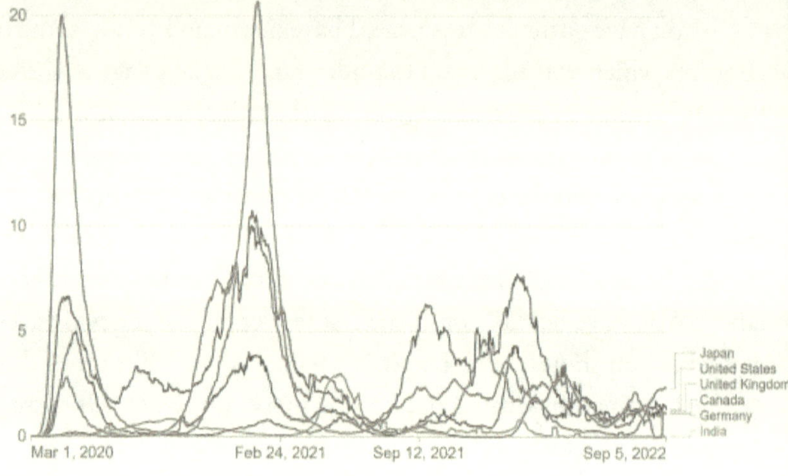

Figure 1

Vaccines available Jan 2021

Nadir July 10 2021

Delta July 10 2021 to Jan 2022

Omicron Jan 2022 to present.

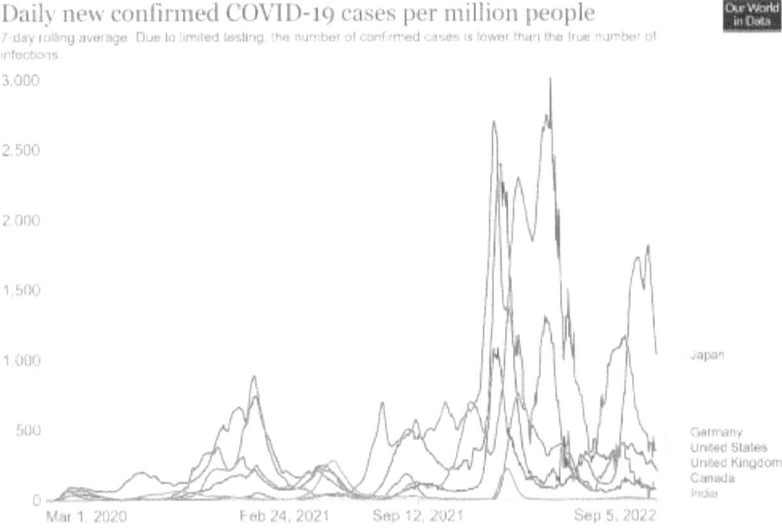

The vaccines appeared to be working after introduction Jan 2021 with a low point about six months later. There followed Delta which was less infective but more virulent. Now we have Omicron which is more infective but less virulent.

Over the last 12 months, this does not appear to be following the normal course of events we have seen in the past. If we had an effective vaccine, the cases should be falling. If we had no treatment, by now, more than two years later, we should see some falling in both cases and deaths.

The longer this continues, the total number of deaths, with mass vaccinations with an ineffective vaccine, may exceed the total number than if we had done nothing.

BACKGROUND

Let's start out by listing some things on which we all agree. The vaccine induces the production of antibodies against the various antigens coded by the mRNA of the spike protein. This is not quite the same as using the whole virus to make the vaccine but seems to be sufficient.

We remember the natural infection involves the interaction of macrophages and dendritic cells with the virion such that the virus can be engulfed, the proteins broken down into 10 amino acid segments, and these segments presented to the surface of cells attached to the MHC molecules. The immune system recognizes the MHC, and then absorbs the antigen attached to begin the formation of cytotoxic T cells and sensitized B cells that make antibodies.

There are lots of antigens as the spike protein contains 1200 amino acids. The spike protein is in two segments, **S1 subunit and S2 subunit**. S1 subunit is the part of the protein that attaches to the receptor. We call this part the N (for nitrogen) terminal domain, **NTD**. The other segment of the protein, S2 subunit, is attached to the body of the virion.

The **NTD, is part of S1** which is about 600 amino acids. This region is next to the part of the spike that connects to the target cell receptor which is called **the receptor binding domain or RBD.** This is that tulip petal I told you about earlier which can be in the open position, meaning it is ready to attach to the receptor on the target cell, or in the closed position, meaning it is bound to one of the other spike proteins. Recall the spike protein is composed of three identical proteins twisted around each other. Hence, we have three petals to this tulip and sometimes one of the petals will be bound (temporarily) to one of the other spikes.

Within the **RBD (receptor binding domain)** is a smaller area called the receptor **binding motif (RBM)**. This is a region comprised of the amino acids that actually attach to the target cell receptor. As soon as this attachment is made several enzymes are activated within both the target cell receptor and the spike protein such that a cleavage area between S1 and S2 is activated so that the stalk can bend to enable attachment of the body of the virus to the cell membrane. There are protein segments that stick out of the cleavage site that attach to the cell membrane and draw the virion to the membrane.

When the body of the virion reaches the target cell membrane, enzymes are activated such that the virus membrane can merge with the cell membrane. We have a mustard seed on a basketball and the seed gets absorbed by the basketball. I would imagine the basketball barely noticed.

But the basketball did notice. When foreign objects enter a cell, they are often engulfed by lysosomes. Chemical signals are initiated which are released outside the cell to attract immune cells. Most of the time the cells take care of this objects without bothering the adaptive part (antibodies) of the immune system.

But this is no normal foreign object. This is a piece of RNA. This is taken by microtubules in the cell to a ribosome where the mRNA is reproduced. If you put mRNA in a ribosome, it just does its job and makes a protein out of it. The viral protein produced stops the signaling of the cell to the immune system, shuts down production of other mRNA, and starts taking over the cells structures to make virions. These virions are transported to the cell membrane and the immune system then does get to recognize them. These virions can also infect neighboring cells. We estimate up to 10 billion virions are made daily by an infected cell. Of these, only about 10,000 are capable of infection.

The mRNA in the vaccine just codes for the spike protein, not for the who virion. With a normal infection, the viral mRNA codes for the entire virus. Many copies of the spike protein are created, but only about one in ten thousand copies develop into functional virions that can go to other cells and infect them. The cell makes lots of spike proteins which are often presented on the cell surface or can be encapsulated and spread throughout the body. These are not complete viruses but rather just spike protein.

The mRNA vaccine was designed to make lots of spike protein, and we want the immune system to identify these proteins and start making antibodies. The vaccine stimulates the presence of about ten times the amount of spike protein as a natural infection would. We now recognize this may be involved in the development of **Long Covid**.

Antibodies attach to the virions and other antigens on the cell surface and signal the immune system to destroy this cell and everything in it. Antibodies attach to the spike protein and keep it from reaching the receptor and infecting the cell to start with. Natural killer t-cells can recognize the antigens on the cell membrane and destroy the cell without any antibody help.

We also all agree the ACE2 receptor is found in more abundance in the upper respiratory tract rather than the lower part of the lungs. In other words, the virus enters you through the nose or mouth, usually gets into the mucous, eventually meets a cell, and then binds to a receptor on the cell (ACE2) to activate entry of the virus into the cell. **The RBM (receptor binding motif)** of the spike protein, just a handful of amino acids (a little more than a handful) starts the whole ball rolling.

Our interest in antibodies revolves around neutralizing antibodies, which are antibodies that prevent the infection of the covid virus. When we check the plasma of those who have recovered from covid, we find many different antibodies to the spike protein. About 80% attach to the RBD part of the stalk and about 20% to the NTB region.

We want antibodies to prevent attachment of covid virus to the receptor on the cell or prevent the virion from attaching to the cell membrane. There are many spots in this area (epitopes) to which the antibodies can bind. The bound antibodies can not only interfere with the binding site, but also change the shape of the site. Remember these proteins are three dimensional. To fit together, the sites must have the right shapes. Just changing the shape may prevent infection.

We have lots of different antibodies (IgG types) that are sensitized to attach to lots of different places on the spike protein, primarily in the **RBD and NTD regions**. Like all our antibodies, the numbers surge with each exposure to the antigens. This occurs not only through repeat vaccine shots or boosters, but also to exposure to the virus. It does not have to be the same variant of covid for us to get this surge of antibodies. The variants are similar enough that the immune system recognizes them.

We like the neutralizing antibodies, but all the different covid antibodies are increased. Both neutralizing and non-neutralizing. Different antibodies can be present that do not inhibit infection. In fact, some antibodies may help the virus infect the cell.

If you get the vaccine, you get lots of different antibodies to the original covid virus coded by the mRNA in the vaccine. Recall there are three other structural proteins in the virion than have antigens. The membrane of the virus has antigens that can get antibodies against them. The envelope has antigens, and the nucleoproteins encapsulating the RNA inside the virus have antigens. These antibodies are not necessarily neutralizing antibodies.

If you have a natural infection, you can get antibodies from these other antigens. You also get antibodies for the spike protein, but the proteins particular to that variant. Many of the antigens of the variants are common to the antigens in the original covid virus, but not all of them. If the cell is making 10 billion virus particles daily (your whole body at the peak of infection) , you would not be surprised if various amino acids were changed, deleted, or even added. Almost all of these mutations serve no purpose to the virus and may actually disable the virus But, if you happen to get one that enables the spike protein to avoid the neutralizing antibodies, then that is the one that will survive the immune pressure of the vaccine antibodies. Those other virions without that mutation will be neutralized while the mutant will survive and prosper. If you happen to get a mutation that enhances infectivity, not only avoiding neutralization but enhancing infection, perhaps by reproducing faster or binding to the receptor better or perhaps merging with the cell wall better, then that virus will outcompete the original virus, dodge the vaccine neutralizing antibodies, and we have a new variant taking over.

For the most part, vaccine neutralizing antibodies will promote inhibition of infection of cells expressing high level of ACE2. These cells are typically found in the upper respiratory tract. This works via antibody mediated hindrance of ACE2 viral entry. The antibodies bind to parts of the RBD, but if you have a mutation to that part and different amino acids are present, the antibody can't find that epitope in order to bind to it.

By now we know that there have been several surges of covid infections around the world. The chart shows what is going on in the United States. It is easy to come to the conclusion that various mutations have occurred that enable the covid virus spike protein to escape the effects of neutralizing antibodies. Monoclonal antibodies were developed using the most potent neutralizing antibodies. These worked for a while, but now are easily shown to be ineffective in some variants such as Omicron. The best antibody against the original spike protein is now not effective. I reviewed the US variants last chapter and now will confine the discussion to Omicron.

Vacinees (those who have been vaccinated with the current vaccines, now about 85% of the adult population) have now become more susceptible to infection. Although their vaccine antibodies are still protecting them somewhat from severe infection, as in death, hospitalizations of fully vaccinated individuals are increasing (see hospitalization chart)

If we had no vaccines or treatment, we would expect a high peak infection and death rate, followed by progressively smaller surges till the epidemic abated, that is herd immunity. We would also see something like this if we had a vaccine that continued to protect from infection. We know this is not the case right now. We are suspicious that mass vaccination is shifting the course of a natural pandemic by promoting the expansion in prevalence of more infectious immune escape variants.

ANTIBODY DEPENDENT ENHANCEMENT OF INFECTION
ADEI

We get the vaccine, and we get a high level of antibodies, both neutralizing and non-neutralizing. The levels the vaccine induces is much higher than a natural infection would, a medium of about 17 times higher. Every time we get a booster or get re-infected, this level goes up, often higher than the initial vaccine. The neutralizing antibodies are not working as well secondary to mutations in the RBD (receptor binding domain) which is keeping these neutralizing antibodies from blocking the RBM (receptor binding motif) from binding the ACE2 (angiotensin 2 converting enzyme) receptor which the covid virus has hijacked, and thus the virus can now enter the cell.

Nevertheless, we keep jacking up the antibodies since a very high level still may have some effectiveness, although that high level doesn't last as long, now only maybe a couple months. We are also jacking up these non-neutralizing antibodies. What about them?

The NTD (N terminal domain) is next door to the RBD. There are separate antibodies to this region. These antibodies bind to epitopes which results in keeping open the petals It so happens this region of the NTD is conserved in the variants, so these antibodies have no trouble binding.

Dr. Bossche, and others, believe that the antibodies to the NTD, which are not neutralizing antibodies, are able to bind to epitopes on the NTD, and as a result of this binding can change the three-dimensional configuration of the intertwined spike proteins. Recall three proteins make up the one stalk of the spike protein. The result of this binding is that they hold the petals in the open position, enabling access of the receptor binding motif (those amino acids that bind to the ACE2 receptor) to the receptor on the cell membrane which enhances the ability of the stalk protein to attach and infect the cell. Elevated levels of neutralizing antibodies also produce elevated levels of non-neutralizing antibodies which bind to the NTD region which promotes the open position of the petals. Every time you get a vaccine, booster, or repeat infection you elevate both types of antibodies which further promotes the open position, which further enhances infectiousness.

The neutralizing antibodies are becoming less and less effective in binding to the variants RBD region, so these elevated levels are inhibiting infection less, while at the same time the other antibodies are enhancing infection. We must keep boosting the antibody levels to try to extend their protective effect. Despite boosting these levels, the variants produce less binding of the neutralizing antibodies so that the protective level must be high to get any protection The antibody levels wane as time goes on. The protective level drops. As the neutralizing antibody becomes less effective, the level required for protection rises. This means the length of time it offers protection drops, now only about 3 months. The non-neutralizing antibodies do not have that problem and they continue to bind without difficulty. We raise them to high levels hence we increase the infectiveness. After a few months the results of higher infectiveness and lower protection result in repeat infections of covid.

This all started with the mRNA vaccines. Ends up the elevated antibody level did not last as long as expected. As they got lower, the neutralizing antibodies did not work as well. This enabled the virus to last longer in the body and drove the development of mutations that were more resistant to the neutralizing effect of the antibody. This led to variants such that the vaccine protected you less against infection. As more people got vaccinated, more people got re-infected, and more people got boosted, the antibody levels kept rising, including the non-neutralizing antibodies, which enhanced the infectiveness of the virus and hence drove the evolutionary dynamics of the virus to more and more infections and less time between recurrent infections.

Recall your innate immune system, the one that initially contacts foreign antigens and formulates IgM, a different type of antibody which is not that specific but responds to initial infection more rapidly. The IgM is around all the time and does not need to wait for IgM to be created. One aspect of the innate immune system is the activation of various interferons. These are chemicals which stimulate many of the components of the immune system. IgM also binds to virions and viral antigens which promotes the destruction of these elements by the rest of the immune system such as NK lymphocytes, neutrophils, dendrite cells, macrophages, and T lymphocytes. This is so efficient that most of the time the antigens do not hang around long enough to stimulate many of the B cell lymphocytes, the cells that turn into antibody producing cells, to make much of a response. In fact, when we give people normal vaccines, we add an adjuvant to get the antigens to hang around longer.

The elevated IgG neutralizing hormones that no longer work well still bind to the spike protein, but now they are obstructing the IgM antibodies from binding to these sites to prevent infection. Hence the antibodies that work cannot bind because the antibodies that don't work are clogging up the antigen sites because we have boosted their levels so high.

You don't get brand new antibodies if you get a variant infection and have previously been vaccinated. The memory cells you developed from the original spike protein get activated and start producing antibodies to that original stalk protein, not to the new variant stalk protein. Your immune system will not go through the trouble of making a new type of IgG if the old antigen is similar enough to the new one. But the innate immune system can form brand new IgM that can recognize and be trained for new antigens, just like the NK lymphocytes can be trained for the new antigens in the variant infections. Of course, your high levels of not very effective neutralizing antibodies and the effective non-neutralizing antibodies are taking up the binding site and inhibiting the training of the innate system. This leads to further susceptibility to infection to those who have been vaccinated. Given what we can observe, that is Omicron is highly infective yet does not seem to produce as severe a disease. Dr. Bossche gives a mechanism by which this can occur.

Remember, the IgM antibodies get elevated and trained during a natural infection. The IgG does not appear for a few weeks. When the IgG starts being produced, the IgM level drops. Every time the IgG level gets boosted, the IgM diminishes.

If you are vaccinated and you happen to get a covid infection, or if you get vaccinated within a couple weeks of infection, your innate immune effector cells may not get the opportunity to develop good immunity. In other words, they do not get trained. It takes several weeks of exposure to train the innate system The vaccine will stimulate elevated levels of IgG against the spike protein which will suppress any IgM production. This is not an unknown phenomenon, and it therefore would not be wise to vaccinate in the middle of a highly infections epidemic. Of course, in this case we did not have a vaccine before the epidemic started and we determined the risk/benefit was in favor of getting vaccinated in the middle of an epidemic. This would have been a good idea if the epidemic acted like other epidemics and the vaccine acted like the usual vaccines. Now we have an almost three ½ year run of the epidemic with no end in sight. We may have burned some of our bridges as far as activating the innate system for training.

Children may have high quantities of innate antibodies, but these are largely naïve. Therefore, if vaccinated, the spike protein antibodies will outcompete the innate antibodies and prevent innate training against covid. In addition, keeping kids home from school and wearing masks, as well as quarantine of healthy children who test positive may inhibit innate immune system sensitization to the normal respiratory viruses children get which mostly result in benign disease. This may result in more severe infections as they get older as the innate system has not been trained.

The adaptive memory system is powerful as it produces copious IgG against specific antigens. The innate system does not have that capacity, and instead sensitizes the cells to varied antigens of the disease and stimulates all the components, NK cells, IgM, interferon, to fight the infection. Even if not completely successful, it reduces the viral load which assists the adaptive system.

Overall, the innate systems are suppressed as we have high vaccination rates in countries. We have a high infection rate which is boosting elevation of non-effective neutralizing antibodies and infection enhancing non neutralizing antibodies. This has resulted in a loss of the ability of the population to develop herd immunity.

-Vaccines are like getting repeat covid infections. This raises the anti-RBD antibodies (the neutralizing antibodies which are not working well) and their anti-NTD antibodies , the antibodies next door to the RBD part of the spike protein which enhance infection.

Dr. G Vanden Bossche DVM, PhD

I have already published the book *Covid and Vaccines for Health Professionals.* In it I do go through every line of the paper inserting the definitions of words, numerous explanatory comments, comments on the contents of the footnotes (generally to show how these relate to the footnoted line in the paper and edit the content to make it easier to read (Dr.Bossche is not a native speaker of the American English language.). The paper appears to have been written to vaccine and viral experts who have an extensive background of the subject.

There is agreement about the first part of Dr. Bossche's paper. The concept of antibody dependent enhancement of infection was known to occur occasionally, but this is the first time during a pandemic. By now you recognize this is much more likely to happen if you have a vaccine that is not sterilizing thus you are not immune from infection if you get the vaccine and are still able to spread the disease and getting the disease does not protect you from reinfection.

If you did not get a covid vaccine, and you get infected, you do seem to have more resistance to another infection for at least a year. If the genome of the virus changes significantly, you will not have as much as your immune system does not recognize that you already had this infection. If your innate immune system is not depressed, you will still be able to rid the body of the virus rapidly.

If you get the covid vaccine, you will boost of your antibodies, but these antibodies will not protect you very long. The antibody boost will make it more likely you will get infected. The repeated elevations of IgG levels will discourage your immune system from creating any different new antibodies to covid variants, as once it has been activated to an antigen, it responds to that antigen (or one similar) and does not begin generating a new different immune response. You are also likely to depress your innate immune system which makes it more likely you will get an infection to start with. We will get more data as time goes on that will enable us to make better decisions, but it does appear that once vaccinated you are stuck with that status.

It is much more controversial as to what is going to happen in the near future. This is the point of the paper.

Currently we now have a highly infectious variant with low virulence(Omicron). Many get infected but few die. We can look at the chart. The number of infections is probably much higher than depicted as many mild infections are not even reported. Many may not even know they had covid. The deaths are probably more accurate. So now the risk of dying from covid (not with covid) is around .1%. It may be lower.

Most of us agree that we can live with this. Most have had the vaccine, but even if you have not, if you are healthy your risk is very low, maybe on the order of .01%. If nothing changes, we will just go on with our lives like before.

Let us look a little closer at the chart. There was a surge in deaths with the Delta variant About Jan 2021 the vaccine began. Deaths and cases dropped till about June 2021. For the next few months, the Delta variant became dominant. You can see how the cases rose and the deaths rose. This was supplanted by the Omicron variant. The cases rose dramatically, and although the total number of deaths were also elevated, the incidence of hospitalization and death fell. There was a slight rise in Feb 2023. We hear people saying the vaccine is working.

But wait a minute. The same antibodies were present during the Delta surge as during the Omicron surge. We now know what is happening. We have discussed ADEI and how it is due to the antibody, the same one present during the Delta. We now know the same antibody raising infectiousness is also decreasing virulence (I will explain this later).

I have mentioned evolutionary dynamics. This is the concept that life will try to reproduce itself. Plants, animals, bacteria, viruses, all will try to reproduce. In fact, they will try to reproduce as much as possible. If the virus of a covid infected person is reproducing a billion virions daily, there will be mutations created. Unless this mutation gives this particular virion some advantage, nothing will come of it. If you have an antibody that can prevent the virion from reproducing or spreading, there will be pressure exerted by the immune system as you are selecting those virions who can resist the antibody to survive. These are the ones that will be used to reproduce. As these virions infect other people, the process will continue to be repeated and each generation will start out with a little better virion in terms of reproduction.

If you have effective neutralizing antibodies, The virus will be eliminated before it has a good chance to evolve. The longer the virus survives in the population, the greater the risk of a resistant variant.

This immune pressure is present with Omicron, but since the vaccine antibodies do not put much immune pressure on the virions, (they are not keeping them from reproducing), it will probably delay the new variant. I say this but there appears to be a new variant that is more infectious that it becomes the dominant variant appearing every few months. If the current booster which contains BA.4 and BA.5 antigens even works a little better than the original vaccine, this will put more immune pressure by the virus to develop a variant that will be resistant to any new antibodies.

Like every other variant, it will probably be more infectious. If the new vaccine produces antibodies that work great (and it will not because these will be the same antibodies we have now), we do not care as it will provide sterilizing neutralization and the virus won't be able to survive enough to spread. By that I mean it will not be able to produce enough virions to spread very easily through the population and thus start approaching herd immunity.

If a new variant does develop and continues to be just as infectious or more, there is no guarantee that it will be less virulent. Let me explain what Dr. Bossche thinks.

You get covid when free virions enter into the mucous of the upper respiratory cavity and encounter the ACE2 receptor on the cell membrane. You have the basketball with a mustard seed bouncing into it (through Brownian motion) and a stalk protein (about one fourth the size of the mustard seed trying to attach to a receptor on the surface (about one eighth the size of the stalk. The non-neutralizing antibodies are holding open the petal on the end of the stalk to make it easier to bind to the receptor. There may be thousands of these virions surrounding this cell, but that would only be a thousand mustard seeds around a basketball.

If you had never gotten the vaccine or never had covid before, you would not have any antibodies around other than non-specific IgM. The virus enters through the upper respiratory tract and eventually makes its way to the respiratory cells. The receptor binding motif (composed of a handful of amino acids) must now connect to the receptor (not an easy task), activate enzymes on the virus and the cell membrane which enables the stalk to attract the viral cell membrane to the respiratory cell membrane and enter the cell. Before that the virion did have to negotiate the innate immune system, which is not that easy.

The virus then enters the cell by activating enzymes which enable the body of the virion to merge with the cell membrane and then either inject the mRNA into the cell or get the cell membrane to engulf the whole virion.

In about three days the virus has started making more virions which go to the surface of the cell to be budded off the cell to infect others.

Recall that your innate immune system has been putting up a fight. IgM is around which can bind to several parts of the virion. This could inhibit the receptors from binding or mark the particle for destruction(opsonization).

The virion can spread through this same process or can infect a neighboring cell without having to go through binding to a receptor. You can see the more receptors, the more likely it is for the cell to get infected.

More severe disease occurs when the virion infects other parts of the body like the lower respiratory tract or more distant organs. These regions may not have many ACE2 receptors and may not have access to as many free virions. It does not appear that covid spreads much through the blood. You can find some evidence of the virus in the blood of those with severe infections, but it is not clear that this is the way the virus spread to these areas.

Enter the dendritic cell. This is the cell that links the innate and the adaptive system. It engulfs virions and presents them to the surface of the cell membrane. It then travels through the lymphatic system as well as the rest of the body. It presents these antigens to various lymphocytes so they can be activated if they contain this antigen. Whole virions can also be attached to these dendritic cells (mustard seeds attached to the basketball cell membrane). and can be carried throughout the body that way and can cause cellular infections if the virion attaches to another cell. In this case the basketball is the dendritic cell, and the mustard seed is attached to the cell membrane, but not infecting the cell.

I am now going to talk about glycoprotcins and how thc connection between high infectiousness of the virus is coupled with low virulence, and how these two characteristics may become disconnected in the covid virus.

We can now perform viral genotyping rapidly and we could identify changes from the original genotype in the areas of the virus responsible for infection. the antibodies to the original genotype were not working as well on the mutated genotypes.

Viruses undergo mutations and there is a natural rate of mutations. Usually these do not necessarily result in a change in virulence or infectiousness, but they sometimes do. We are now undergoing a rapid rate of mutations in the covid virus, and they seemed to be concentrated in a certain portion of the spike protein. Again, not the usual scenario.

When a virus becomes widespread, that used to mean it has developed a mutation that allows it to outcompete all the other viruses. It has already been honed by nature and is now the fittest.

It's like the bacterial gut biome. You have many microbes in your gut that survive and thrive. In fact, many provide a health benefit for you. It's as if the bacteria have been created to keep you alive, or more accurately allow you to extract nutrients from your food, such that the bacteria always have a place to live. This is now a stable environment as the competition among other bacteria has enabled the survival of the fittest, which includes keeping you healthy.

Sure, there are mutations, but these mutations must provide some benefit in order for them to become the dominant species in that niche. Things don't change unless we do something like take antibiotics that allows another bacterium that can adapt to the antibiotics to take over. It could not take over unless you changed things. Not only antibiotics, but there are hundreds of chemicals in our environment you ingest, chemicals that may not have existed 150 years ago may allow these bacteria to thrive.

We now can document many mutations in the spike protein. These enabled that variant to outcompete the other variants and become dominant for a short period of time, only to be replaced by a new variant.

We have lots of antibodies from vaccines and re-exposure to the covid virus through mild infections or boosters. But as Dr. Bossche has explained, the neutralizing antibodies against the spike protein (those developed against the original spike protein) are becoming progressively less effective. It now appears the non-neutralizing antibodies may be increasing the infectiousness of virus, the opposite of what we used to expect a vaccine to do. It's an endless circle as we get a booster which increases the antibodies from the original vaccine which increases the antibodies that make the virus more infective which makes us catch the virus again.

Our CDC has been wrong in their predictions of the evolutionary dynamics of covid. I simply do not trust them to know what is going on. Of course, they will never admit they may have been wrong, which is odd because it they did that, I may trust them more. Dr. Bossche is going predict what will most likely happen, based not upon guessing or what he wants to be true, but "following the science".

I have heard that we were funding gain of function for this virus. That means we were changing the genome to make the SARS-Cov-1 virus more infective. That is something we used to do so we could develop future vaccines against a virus. Not a completely crazy thing to do but perhaps a little risky. My intuition tells me this virus escaped from the Wuhan lab, probably by accident but I am not sure.

Now adays it may be crazy to do gain of function. It only takes a few months to develop an mRNA vaccine. We can find out the genotype of a virus in a few days. This may explain why this virus is vulnerable to so many mutations in a particular region of the stalk protein, which is the receptor Binding Domain (RBD)

I have written the book *Covid and Vaccines for Medical Professionals* in which I reviewed a paper by Dr. Bossche regarding his predictions as to the outcome of the covid epidemic. In the next chapters I will go over the general outline as to how he reached this conclusion. For more details you can get the above book or actually read the paper itself.

PAPER

Poor virus-neutralizing capacity in highly C-19 vaccinated populations could soon lead to a fulminate spread of SARs-CoV-2 super variants that are highly infections and highly virulent in vaccinees while being fully resistant to all existing and future spike-based C-19 vaccines. Geert Vanden Bossche DVD, PhD, voiceforscienceandsolidarity.org

https://uploads-ssl.webflow.com/ 616004c52e87ed08692f5692/ 627933433cc6dc1c869df8ad_GVB%27s%20analysis%20of%20C-19%

One of the goals of this book is to present the predictions of this paper such that you can have an understanding of the covid epidemic and the vaccines that have been created. The new mRNA vaccines are not the same as our previous vaccines. It is progressively evident that the immunologic response to the vaccine is not the same as one would get with a natural infection, or with the previous vaccine strategy we have used for the last 100 years.

Dr. Bossche predicts what may happen. Now it may not happen but, for you to understand the concept I had to teach you some information so you could use you common sense and understand the language.

The previous book was *Covid and Vaccines for Medical Professionals* in which I went through the paper line by line giving some definitions and explanatory comments along the way. I did include the contents of this book. You can always read the paper yourself but unless you are quite familiar with the language of virology and immunology it will be a difficult read. The paper was written to those who are practicing in that field. I will give a summation of his argument in the next few chapters.

I have laced this book with some of my opinions. It should be evident what are my thoughts and what are those of Dr. Bossche. You of course will not agree with all that I say, but at least you will think about it and come up with a better opinion, which if I think are better than mine, I will soon incorporate it in the book as the paperback books are printed on demand and I can change the contents in about one day. Like all my books I am interested in teaching you something.

Dr. Bossche goes into great detail in his 45-page paper to explain what happened. What follows is my summation.

I have already gone over the concept of antibody dependent enhancement of infection in the previous chapter. It is important you see this as it is critical the understanding of the dynamics of the relationship of the mRNA vaccine in the mechanisms of the epidemic. This is not a new concept and has been seen in other diseases, but not really other epidemics. Upon reading more about the vaccine, this was actually mentioned as a possibility, but it was discounted as being unlikely. Now it is integral to our present state. Dr. Bossche goes over this in the first part of the paper.

Another concept repeatedly mentioned is evolutionary dynamics. Let me be clear, I believe man, all life, all the earth, and all the universe is created by God. Once the book, Origin of the Species became popular, this hijacked the meaning of evolution to mean man was not created. A description of the reproduction of the virus could also me called population dynamics, but evolutionary dynamics is the term used by the paper.

There are about 8 billion people on the earth. This is about the same number of virions produced by a person during a covid infection. In order to produce these your body must put together at least 1200 amino acids (the length of the spike protein) Usually your body does a great job turning DNA into RNA but translating this RNA (or any other RNA such as the RNA you got from getting infected by an RNA virus) into proteins may contain errors. As such, you get many versions of the RNA which may not be identical. Sometimes you skip an amino acid, sometimes you change one, sometimes they are in a different order. Most of the time even these slightly abnormal proteins that are produced will still work, just maybe not as well.

If one of these abnormal infectious virions is lucky enough to infect another cell in your body, that infected cell will then produce many copies of this virion. If you infect someone else with covid, all the virions produced by that person will contain this abnormal RNA.

All life is driven to reproduce. Otherwise as time goes on that life would cease to exist. This is true of all microorganisms, plants , and animals. All reproduction contains the possibility of passing an abnormal protein along to its offspring. It does not take long for microorganisms to take over an environment. The gut biome is a good example. You have many more cells (bacterial) in your gut than you do in the rest of your body. They are all reproducing. Many exist in a certain environment that may be constantly changing. If you take antibiotics for a couple weeks, the bacteria of a certain species that are less susceptible to that antibiotic will increase in population as they will be able to reproduce better. We call this evolutionary dynamics, which is the ability to adapt to a different biome.

This is simplified in viral infections as we are dealing with a much smaller amount of DNA or RNA. If an infectious virion is made that infects another cell in your body and there is a mutation around which makes it slightly more resistant to antibodies present, the other cells infected with that virion will resist the antibiotic better and hence may survive longer and therefore produce more of these virions. There will then be a better chance that the virions that have this mutation will be the ones that infects someone else.

Viral mutations happen all the time, but unless it gives some advantage, in this case we are talking about becoming more infectious, it will not take over the biome. So even if the virion that infected you is not exactly like the virion that infected your neighbor, it will not become dominant unless it becomes more infective. Now that doesn't mean it may not make you a little sicker or cause a little different symptom, but it will not take over.

If this mutation is deadlier and more likely to kill you, it will still not take over unless it is more infective. It is possible that a virus may get a mutation that gets the cell to produce more virions and hence spread a little better, but it appears for covid the bottom line for becoming the dominant virus is to be able to resist the antibodies. That results in a longer infection which gives a longer time to spread the virus, and also results in initial resistance to the adaptive immune system which means the innate system is not getting any help. The innate system will eventually win (if it doesn't you will die), but it may take longer which mean more viral spread, and more reproductive cycles of the virus.

You get exposed to the covid virus, but most people do not develop an infection. That means your immune system is able to suppress and eliminate the virus. Most of the time this is what happens to all viruses you are exposed to. Some have become dominant such as they are able to subvert the innate system for long enough that they can spread. If you are unvaccinated, you get infected because your innate system did not eliminate the virus fast enough. If the virus hangs around long enough, your adaptive system kicks in to make antibodies which greatly aids in viral elimination.

If you had a normal vaccine, your innate system gets help within a few days which hastens the complete elimination of the virus before a functional infection can occur. Thus, you have no symptoms (or very few), and the virus is not spread.

For reasons previously mentioned, we now have less than effective neutralizing antibodies. Remember if the concentration of antibodies is very high, it will provide neutralization of the virus and help the innate system such that no infection results after exposure. For this vaccine this effect is only working for 2-3 months as the antibody level drops. For a real vaccine the antibody level remains high enough for years, thus effecting herd immunity,

After a few months, the antibody levels are not high enough to prevent infection. Hence if the innate system cannot prevent infection rapidly enough, you will get a more widespread covid infection which lasts a relatively long time. Now in most people, your innate system eventually wins as the death rate is low (the present variants are less than .1%) But the lack of effectiveness results in longer infections which results in more replication cycles of the virus which results in a greater production of possible mutations.

But that is not all. Like bacterial infections in which antibiotics are selecting out the bacteria that are resistant to those antibiotics, antibodies which are not highly effective are slowly selecting out those mutations which allow the cells infected with covid to survive the antibodies. This is what drives evolutionary dynamics. It is a numbers game.

Covid vaccination results in loads of covid antibodies. That is not the problem. Now covid antibodies result in increased risk of infection secondary to ADEI. We have higher risk of infection, antibodies that are not rapidly helping the innate system to stop the infection, and these same antibodies selecting out the cells which are producing more infectious variants. We are promoting mutations.

Let's look a little deeper. Dr. Bossche does not mention this, but it is possible the virus itself may have been genetically manipulated to produce a higher mutation rate than a natural virus.

Now back to mRNA. It may be likely the vaccine itself may produce a diminution in the effectiveness of the innate system by adversely affecting interferon production. I already discussed how the rapid rise in IgG from vaccination inhibits the training of the innate system further decreasing its effectiveness. These same IgG antibodies both inhibit production of IgM from the innate system, and also diminish their actions by physically preventing their attachment to epitopes on the stalk protein.

Now the good news. You are still winning. Sure, more people may get infected, but it is only a small percentage of the population. Even then, few people are dying. I agree herd immunity is no closer than ever, but if we look at the situation objectively, more damage was done by government actions against the pandemic than the pandemic itself.

Your immune system is quite potent, and your body has numerous mechanisms to protect you from disease.

So, why worry? That is the second half of Dr. Bossche's paper.

PAPER PART TWO

If we look at the CDC charts, there is obviously a relationship between the increased infections, yet the lower death rate. Some will consider this to be a blessing as more people get covid yet do not die from it. With a normal viral infection such as influenza, after catching the infection and not dying, you would then usually be immune to further infection. It is a natural vaccine.

As we understand now, this is not the case. Still there is some mechanism by which the antibodies that enhance infection also diminish disease. Covid initially infects the upper respiratory tract. Severe disease is related to lower respiratory tract infection and lung infection appears to be the gateway for appreciable viremia (virions found in the blood) which is associated with %100 of the patients in the ICU) Infection in the upper respiratory tract results from virions passing through the mucous and having direct contact with the epithelial cell. For the cell to be easily infected it must have the ACE2 receptor on the cell membrane.

I have earlier described what happens next. It ends up that the cell membrane must also express the TMPRESS2 protein on the membrane, which is the enzyme that separates the S1 and S2 units of the stalk protein and allows the virion to merge and enter the cell. The lungs appear to play a large factor in the progression to severe disease.

The virus then propagates down the airways (bronchioles), perhaps by infecting the ciliated cells there. This seems to produce a more robust innate immune response. This makes sense as your upper respiratory system cells are continuously exposed to various infective agents. Almost all the time the local innate system prevents infection. Should the infection start to propagate, now you get the immune systems attention. If you remember your anatomy, the sacs in the lung, that is the alveoli, allow oxygen to pass from the airways into the bloodstream. In other words, it is somewhat like the skin in the sense it separates the outside environment from the inside of your body. Unlike the skin, this is a thin membrane so your body must be vigilant to keep pathogens from using this entry point to get into your bloodstream.

Most of the time (> than 99% for omicron) the disease is confined to the upper respiratory tract, but some progress to infect cells in the alveoli. These are called type II pneumocytes. This leads to more severe disease. This is what we see in those who die, an adult respiratory distress syndrome in which the death of the pneumocytes leads to an immune reaction in which fibrin and aberrant healing is present.

The key to diminishing the death rate is to interrupt the progression to the pneumocytes. Dr Bossche explains how the antibodies which enhance infection of the Omicron variant also reduces the infection of these pneumocytes.

At this point let me put things in perspective. As of today in the US, we have had about one hundred million cases (probably more) and one million deaths (probably a little less as dying with covid and from covid is a gray area) We know that some of these high-risk patients may have died anyway. There is also some controversy over whether the covid vaccine itself may be inducing excess death. I am going to say about 1% of those with covid died. Keep in mind that this has been over more than three years. The current death rate from the Omicron variant is much less.

Let's say the population of the US is 300 million This means about .3% of the population died from covid. With the Spanish Flu. It is estimated about 1% of the population died from that. The significance of Dr. Bossche's paper is his prediction of a more serious variant, which is one more infectious and virulent, and the interaction of this with the current vaccines.

The death rate off the original SARS-CoV-1 (about 20 years ago) was almost 10%. This variant was not nearly as infective as SARS

CoV-2, but obviously more virulent. If would not be hard to imagine a more virulent version of the present virus.

The dendritic cell plays an important role in expressing antigens to the adaptive immune system such that antibodies can be developed. It is the connection between the innate and adaptive system. It expresses antigens on both the MHC-1 complexes to cytotoxic lymphocytes and MHC-2 complexes to B and T lymphocytes. In doing so it is a motile cell which travels throughout the body.

When the dendritic cell encounters a covid virion which is not attached to an antibody, this virion can attach itself to the cell membrane of the dendritic cell. Recall our basketball with the mustard seed attached (this is an approximate image but pretty close) The virion attaches and travels around on the basketball. Many cells in your body move around and bump into other cells. The T and B lymphocytes must bump into other cells to get the antigens attached to the MHC complexes. These complexes are about the size of a receptor, yet the cells manage to get close enough to almost touch the cell membrane. You have a receptor on the dendritic cell which is smaller than a mustard seed hooking up with another basketball with a particle smaller than a mustard seed attached to it in order to transfer the antigen. It seems unlikely that this could happen but in small particles forces like electrostatic attraction have a significant effect.

Lectins are proteins found on the surface of the cell membrane of dendritic cells as well as on all kinds of cells. These proteins are called lectins because they bind to carbohydrate structures, which as you know are called glycans. We know that the spike protein has glycans all over the 1200 amino acid stalk.

At this point you may be asking yourself "why do these cells have these things."? The cell membrane is quite dynamic, and things are always being excreted from the cell or absorbed into the cell. There are receptors all over the cell. In order for absorption or contact with a receptor to be made, things need to be held still for a very short time. The lectins tether another particle to the cell to see if it wants to interact. The covid stalk protein has these glycans and can attach to lectins.

The cell membrane has a slight negative charge. You could see if you made part of the stalk protein have a slight positive charge, it would help the stalk to briefly attach to a receptor to enable activation of enzymes which would begin the infective process of getting the virion into the cell. Certain mutations could change amino acids on the NTD such that it would become more positive and possibly increase the chance of attaching to a receptor. This has been measured and does occur. There is a sweet spot in that if it became too positive, it prevents the virion from being absorbed. It keeps it attached to the membrane.

The virion becomes attached to the dendritic cell via lectins on the surface attaching to glycans on the virion. The lectin was designed to attach to things that the cell might need, but the virion has hijacked the lectin. Just like it uses the receptor for ACE2 to get into the cell.

When the dendritic cell encounters covid virions at the portal of entry, it can engulf these virions and become activated. This means it processes the antigen and presents them on MHC complexes. It then travels throughout the body. Virions not attached to antibodies can then tether themselves to the cell membrane of the dendritic cell. These are virions capable of infection and thus can travel elsewhere, such as the lower respiratory tract, and lead to more severe disease.

As I mentioned before, the cells in the lower respiratory tract have fewer ACE2 receptors so even if the virion arrives, it is more difficult to infect the cells there (type 2 pneumocytes)

There are structures within the bilayer of the cell membrane called lipid rafts. These are small microdomains composed of various lipids and cholesterol, and these rafts seem be linked with the regulation of membrane protein trafficking and often associated with receptors. It appears that the tethering of the virion to the lectin of the membrane of the dendritic cell exposes part of a glycan free zone on the NTD which enables attachment of the NTD to a lipid raft on a target cell membrane. This is another example of the virus hijacking a normal cellular process which is normally used to enable stabilization of a protein (in this case the stalk protein) near a receptor to activate the receptor, but now is using this to enable infection. Without this process it would be much more difficult for the virion to interact with one of these sparse receptors.

This process is called trans infection, which is infection of a cell by virions caried on the dendritic cell. Cells can also be infected by trans fusion. That is the infection of a neighboring cell without requiring an ACE2 receptor. This is especially important in cells that have rare expression of the ACE2 receptor.

The above paragraphs are describing the course of trans infection in someone who does not have any antibodies, that is no vaccine and no natural infection. Even then, the incidence of death from infection, which means the infection has spread throughout the body, is low, on the order of 1-3% (in high-risk people) for the original virus. Your innate system is still working fine.

Let's say you were once infected and now have functioning antibodies, which is neutralizing antibodies which can bind to the RBD of the stalk and prevent attachment of the RBM to the cell ACE2 receptor. First you don't get infected. Second, the antibodies attach to virions that prevents attachment of the virions to the lectin on the dendritic cell. Finally, it prevents any attached virions to dendritic cells from binding to the rare receptors in the lower respiratory tract. We get what we expected, that is we don't get infected and even if this happens, we do not get a severe infection.

We are dealing with populations. Biological processes are not perfect. Even with an ideal antibody it is possible that a rare person may get infected and die. Even with a great vaccine, if you have a defect or weakness in your immune system, you may get infected. But that is not the point. The goal is to prevent an epidemic through herd immunity, and we do not have to be perfect to get that to happen. Just get enough people to the point that the virus can no longer propagate through the population and thus prevent large numbers from dying.

Now we have high levels of ineffective anti-RBD antibodies which does not prevent infection. The high levels of anti-NTD antibodies which go up at the same time promotes infection by inducing an open expression of the RBM and hence facilitates attachment to the ACE2 receptor which lead to infection. This happens secondary to the NTD antibodies inducing conformational changes in the RBD. That is, it changes the arrangement of the proteins such that the RBM remains open. Thus, high levels of infection. But we do not have high levels of death.

It appears these same antibodies that promote an open configuration inhibits attachment of the RBD region to the receptor if the virion is tethered to the dendritic cell. When the virion is tethered to the dendritic cell via the NTD on the stalk protein, the configuration of the region changes. That is not surprising and if there were no antibodies around, it may promote attachment of the tethered virions to the rare ACE2 receptors.

But we have high levels of antibodies. It appears the binding of the anti-NTD antibodies to the changed conformation of the NTD region as a result of tethering to the lectin on the dendritic cell membrane now promotes a closed RBM instead of an open one. This seems to markedly reduce the ability for these tethered virions to produce infection. Hence, we have what we have now, high infections in the upper tract, low in the lower tracts, lower severe disease, and low deaths.

This is good news in that it promotes few deaths and illnesses. I write books on Diet and Health with that goal. I guess we can call our present situation pseudo herd immunity. This is not real herd immunity, but it is better than nothing.

PAPER PART THREE

If we look at evolutionary dynamics, I think I can say the goal of any infectious virus is to create an epidemic. Similarly, the goal of herd immunity is to prevent an epidemic. No matter how you look at it, we currently have an epidemic and hence do not have herd immunity. The virus is winning, and the immune system has not accomplished its goal. You can try to make a deal with the virus, but it is driven to reproduce and will continue to change.

I've heard people say the virus has given us the equivalent of herd immunity. The point of the paper by Dr. Bossche is that it has not. The mass-vaccination campaign did not give us real immunity, and Omicron has not given us real herd immunity. Now we are at the point in the paper that concerns what is next.

You understand how we got to where we are now You understand that our current antibodies are not eliminating the virus. Evolutionary dynamics is forcing the virus to reproduce itself more efficiently, which translates into higher infectiousness. We have lots of people vaccinated which means we have lots of antibodies against the virus. Although not very effective, the high levels of neutralizing antibodies do seem to suppress infection for a few months. They will not sterilize the virus; hence mutations are continuously created. If the mutation either provides resistance to the antibody or produces some other mechanism that increases infectiousness, that version will gradually become the dominant variant.

Some have contended that a virus will never become so deadly that it kills everyone. I agree and that has never happened. But that is not what we are talking about. If the virus killed twenty percent of the people, I don't think that amount would reduce the mutation rate or the development of new variants or reduce its infectivity. Yet it would make a big difference to the living standards of the world. Dr. Bossche, nor really anyone else, thinks that Covid is going to be the end of the world.

What Dr. Bossche does believe is that the mass vaccination of the mRNA vaccine has prevented herd immunity. He believes more infective variants will develop, and probably more virulent viruses.

The various mutations can be identified by doing viral genotyping, which we can now do in a few days. We can look at these and come up with a reason they may cause virulence. We could not look at the genotype and predict the anti-NTD antibodies would cause antibody dependent enhancement of infection.

If we look at the amino acids, we can predict which ones may be susceptible to O-glycosylation or N-glycosylation, but we don't know which glycan may attach to that amino acid or what will be the effect if any,

The glycans that attach to the amino acids on the stalk proteins are made by your own DNA. Glycans are necessary for life and many different ones are made all the time. Viruses can use some of your self-glycans to try to hide from the immune system. Glycan receptors are one way the immune system identifies you from something else.,

There are several factors that determine if a glycan will attach. We already know there are only 3-4 amino acids that attach them. If you get a mutation that changes an amino acid, you may lose a glycan or you may gain one, or you may change one.

The conformation of the protein (stalk) itself may allow certain glycans to attach but not others. Visualize the protein in three dimensions. It can be twisted or folded or not allow enough space for a glycan to attach. The glycans themselves may change things such that a new one may not allow the proper space for an old on.

The anti NTD antibodies currently allow greater infection of the virion, so the virus is not motivated to change that. At the same time, the same antibody prevents spreading of the infection in the body, so logically a mutation that keeps the petals open, but changes the NTD region such that the antibodies will not prevent trans infection is desirable for the virus.

One reasonable way for this to occur is through glycans binding to sites on the NTD that would change the conformation of the stalk. Currently the tethered virions have changed the conformation of the NTD such that attachment closes the petals when it is tethered to the dendritic cell. If not attached, the conformation of the NTD is different such that the same antibody promotes open petals. It is the same genotype but a different conformation. The conformation can also be changed by adding glycans.

You could have an amino acid mutation that allows a glycan to attach to the NTD but does not affect the ability of the antibody to keep the petals open, which continues the ability of the virus to bind to the receptor, just like it does now. But once that conformation has been changed by tethering, that same glycan may allow, or even promote, infection of distant sites. This would obviously be of some advantage to the virus in terms of population dynamics as it would result in a higher level of infectious virions in the host and hence greater infectiousness. This would be a mutation that evolutionary dynamics demands.

There is no reason that at the same time an additional mutation may produce more rapid infection in the upper respiratory tract. You may say it would be crazy for the virus to become deadlier because it would kill the host. But not before it created many more infective virions which would have translated into more infections.

This will have to be a random event but is has been estimated that worldwide there are about 10,000 possible single base mutations a day,

https://www.ncbi.nlm.nih.gov/pmc/articles/PMC7685332/

Total number and mass of SARS-COV-2 virions

Dr. Bossche goes into much more detail as the probable glycosylation that may occur. He also predicts that these glycan alterations may also make the current vaccine generated antibiotics ineffective. Elevated levels will no longer protect you,

I have taught you a lot of information which will enable you to use your common sense in evaluating what you hear in the medical news, from the CDC, and from media outlets. In the last few chapters I will explain what I think you should do now. Let me remind you I am a retired physician and no longer practicing medicine, so nothing I say should be considered medical advice. What I have taught you thus far is not really advice, but rather instruction in the subject of covid and vaccines. Most would agree with the information, although there still may be many who say I am crazy.

WHY

The pandemic was upon us, and we had no vaccine or treatment. If we did nothing, we would expect it to follow the pattern for other epidemics, that is a series of peaks cases and deaths which would get progressively smaller till herd immunity had been reached. We expected that those who recovered from the illness would be immune from further infections. We expected we could decrease the deaths if we had effective treatment. Since, like other epidemics, the old and immune compromised were at increased risk, it would be wise to protect them. We are hoping that enough younger, healthy people will get the diseases, survive, and become immune. Once enough people became immune, herd immunity would be able to protect those at the most risk.

No matter what, there would be many deaths. No one knew how many, but with the Spanish Flu epidemic, this amounted to about 1% of the population in the US. Of course, this was 100 years ago before antibiotics were available to treat secondary pneumonia, so we expected we could lower that percentage.

We placed our faith in a new technology using messenger RNA as a method to provide the immune system with antigens against the virus so that your body could develop protective antibodies against the virus without having to become infected with the virus. Vaccines had worked in the past to avoid as many people dying, yet still achieving herd immunity, and we expected this new vaccine to be no different.

A massive effort was put forth and in one year a vaccine was developed and manufactured to use on the public, not only in the United States but around the world. Several were developed but all relied on mRNA to present spike protein antigens to the immune system. Initially this vaccine worked quite well, and we expected to conquer the pandemic within a year.

After a few months we realized something was not quite right. People were getting infected despite having received the vaccine. In the last few years, we have developed techniques that enable us to map the genotype of a virus.

We can decipher the mRNA and understand the amino acid structure. We used these techniques to build the vaccine. We were now using them to determine that the original mRNA in the virus was changing through mutations. This was rendering the antibodies developed using the original mRNA somewhat less effective.

Around the world there were patterns of the cases and deaths initially decreasing, then surges in both which we were able to determine were due to mutations in variants which were more resistant to the antibodies. Several different variants produced their own spikes. The Delta variant was more virulent causing a greater percentage of deaths, the Omicron variant was more infectious but not as virulent. Despite the fact that the same antibody derived from the original covid was present.

Getting a vaccine did not prevent disease.

Getting the disease did not prevent getting the disease again.

More than two years after the vaccines were distributed, we are not closer to herd immunity.

This does not look like past epidemics.

The key factor in our current situation is the lack of development of sterilizing immunization with the vaccine. The innate immune system can protect against infection and eliminate pathogens, but if this system is unable to eliminate antigens, the adaptive system is a powerful tool. Copious amounts of antibodies to specific antigens can virtually eliminate these antigens through mechanisms described. (Mainly by identifying infected cells and virions to enable their destruction) This results in sterilization (removal of antigens) and activation of antibody production should they reoccur. In other words, you get cured of the infection, you cannot infect anyone, and you do not get re-infected as any repeat exposure to the virus results in its elimination.

Everyone agrees the mRNA vaccine generated many spike protein antigens and enabled your adaptive immune system to mount copious antibodies to these antigens. This seems like the same process that occurs with previous epidemics in which herd immunity developed. What happened?

Dr. Bossche has presented the reason which most people accept. The antibodies did not sterilize the virus. Initially they seemed to be working, but variants developed that became more resistant to the antibodies through mutations. We know that high levels of IgG suppress the innate system somewhat to that specific antigen. If the antibodies do not work as well, and remember this is relative, a high level may be somewhat effective but as this level drops, and normally it does after a few months, they may be less effective, especially if the antigen sites are changing such that the antibodies do not attach as well.

He has explained how the dynamics of evolution means that as these virions are manufactured by infected cells, there will be mutations that occur that change the amino acids in parts of the spike protein such that antibodies do not work. These virions will survive better than the original spike proteins, which are affected by antibodies and hence do not infect as well. The less affected-by-antibodies virions will eventually be the ones that spread to other people, and we now have a new variant. Almost everyone agrees this has happened.

We have gone over the concept of antibody enhancement of infection. This was not an unknown concept but not common and probably not involved in previous epidemics. This can explain our current picture of surges in the number of cases as time goes on, not what we expect in an epidemic.

Again, this is consistent with evolutionary dynamics as this promotes the spread of the virion. The more infectious, the more people get infected, the more virions.

The vaccinal antibodies are now doing the opposite of what we desire. We have antibodies against the RBD, the receptor binding domain, which are supposed to be neutralizing the ability of the virus to enter the cell, but now do not identify these antigens secondary to mutations in this area, and hence are not neutralizing the virus. At the same time, we have non-neutralizing antibodies to the NTD, the N terminal Domain, which is next door to the RBD, which is making it easier for the virus to infect cells. Every time we get re-vaccinated or get exposed to the virus or get infected by the virus, we boost both of these two sets of antibodies. The neutralizing antibodies are working less well as time goes on, the non-neutralizing antibodies are working quite well to enhance infection. This also explains the graphs of cases.

The Delta variant was more virulent (caused greater sickness) than the Omicron. Delta caused a higher death rate, but this variant was overcome by Omicron's high infectiousness. We now have more cases but a lower incidence pf deaths. This also explains the current graphs.

We just went over why the connection between a more infectious, yet less virulent variant has now become dominant. He explains how the very antibodies which increase infection also discourage systemic infection and thus prevent severe illness. This makes some sense and explains the current graphs.

I have explained **WHY** we are in our current state. I will next explain **WHAT HAPPENED**, I will then address **WHAT IS GOING TO HAPPEN.**

WHAT HAPPENED

Why did this happen? I will go over the three main reasons why we are where we are.

We first must look at the virus. This is not acting the way we expected. It was quite infectious from the beginning, spreading around the world in a matter of months. I know in our present society we are quite mobile, and it does not take much for the entire world to get exposed, but even then, it was a rapid expansion. We get a case in the state of Washington or California, and a month later there are cases throughout the US. A few months later it was throughout the world.

This is a genetically modified virus. We know it was from Wuhan, we know it was in the virology lab there, we are pretty certain there were experiments on gain of function of the virus there. We are also somewhat confident that the US was financing the viral modifications. We suspect that the viral security at the laboratory was less than ideal.

I am not sure at all why this has not been well investigated by the US, although if we were paying for this research, I can see how no one is interested in investigating. I am sure that at this point there is no record at all in the Chinese laboratory that this virus was ever there and probably no one involved is there anymore.

I am not a viral expert, but I can see there is a substantial change in the genotype of SARS 1 the SARS 2 virus relating to the amino acids between subunit 1 and subunit 2. If you wanted to make the virus more infective, this is where you would make the modifications. It is difficult for me to believe that this change occurred between the SARs-1 and SARS-2 without any known intervening steps in the natural virus.

It is also not acting like a normal virus. Although the mRNA vaccine has its own problems, we do know that it promoted antibodies against the spike protein. We do know these antibodies were initially effective. We also know that they did not produce a sterilizing condition, which is prevent infection once vaccinated.

We know the main reason was probably the rapid development of variants that were resistant to the neutralizing antibodies secondary to mutations. If the antibody does not cause sterilization, the virus lingers longer in the body, the virus continues to produce more virions, and the antibodies are promoting through immune pressure those spike proteins which are resistant to those antibodies that would produce sterilization.

This process is appearing to occur much more rapidly than previous infectious viruses. Is this a coincidence or is this because this is not a normally evolved virus but one that has been intentionally genetically modified. It may be that even if it was modified the rapid rate of mutations was not intended, but never the less it is there.

Throughout we have been treating this as a normal virus and are surprised when our normal procedures to fight the virus are not working. Perhaps this is the reason why. Did we ever consider this virus was genetically modified and our normal actions had to be modified?

At this point it does not matter, and we deal with what we have. But it may be wise to change our normal approach.

Now let us look at the mRNA vaccine. We keep calling it a vaccine, but it does not act at all like a typical vaccine in the sense that it does not stop you from getting infected.

We all remember the CDC. Get the vaccine to keep from getting infected and eventually establish herd immunity which will make the pandemic go away.

Then it was get the vaccine to protect you grandmother.

Then it was get the vaccine to keep from dying from covid.

Of course, that last one is somewhat true as you realize from reading the paper. At least it is true right now, but perhaps not in the future.

We now are advised to give the vaccine to everyone who has been born prior to the last six months. Dr. Bossche goes in detailed reasoning why this is a terrible idea. I agree.

You got the vaccine, but nobody told you that you don't get something for nothing. This is a new type of vaccine, and it is not the same as the old type.

Now let us look at the vaccine. Look at this paper:

Innate immune suppression by SARS-CoV-2 mRNA vaccinations: The role of G-quadruplexes, exosomes, and MicroRNAs

Stephanie Seneff, Greg Nigh, Anthony M Kyriakopoulos, and Peter A. MCullough

Food Chem Toxicol. 2022 Jun;164: 113008

https://www.ncbi.nlm.nih.gov/pmc/articles/PMC9012513/#bib78

Abstract

The mRNA SARS-CoV-2 vaccines were brought to market in response to the public health crises of Covid-19. The utilization of mRNA vaccines in the context of infectious disease has no precedent. The many alterations in the vaccine mRNA hide the mRNA from cellular defenses and promote a longer biological half-life and high production of spike protein.

However, the immune response to the vaccine is very different from that to a SARS-CoV-2 infection. In this paper, we present evidence that vaccination induces a profound impairment in type I interferon signaling, which has diverse adverse consequences to human health. Immune cells that have taken up the vaccine nanoparticles release into circulation large numbers of exosomes containing spike protein along with critical microRNAs that induce a signaling response in recipient cells at distant sites.

We also identify potential profound disturbances in regulatory control of protein synthesis and cancer surveillance. These disturbances potentially have a causal link to neurodegenerative disease, myocarditis, immune thrombocytopenia, Bell's palsy, liver disease, impaired adaptive immunity, impaired DNA damage response and tumorigenesis.

We show evidence from the VAERS database supporting our hypothesis. We believe a comprehensive risk/benefit assessment of the mRNA vaccines questions them as positive contributors to public health.

The authors conclude that that the immune results of the vaccine are different from those induced by infection. They demonstrate numerous changes that indicate the mRNA vaccine may be doing more harm than good. Especially since now we see the failure of the covid vaccine.

I do recommend you read the article although some "fact checkers" have criticized it. Since the initial publication of this book the paper appears to be accurate. The paper is another example of the suppression of information criticizing the mRNA vaccine. As we are finding out more about Long Covid, the paper rings true.

This book is discussing Dr. Bossche's paper and his predictions of the evolutionary course of covid as it is related to the covid vaccine. I anticipate numerous adverse events will begin to appear as a result of the mRNA vaccine. Over the last year this has happened.

Earlier I mentioned the excess deaths now noted in several countries in which mass vaccination was popular. It is possible this is a result of impaired immunity as mentioned in the abstract. There are several countries who now recognize this occurrence.

Finally, we have mass vaccinations. I remember when the vaccine came out. I read about it and watched videos. I do not recall at all anyone mentioning that instead of just viral mRNA being injected into people, that it was genetically modified mRNA. Now the developers say this was all done to make the vaccine work better, at least their definition of working better, but no one ever mentioned the modifications. These do not appear to be completely benign, and now this may be beginning to manifest itself. Did anyone tell you that the antibody levels induced by the vaccine are 17 time higher than those from a natural infection? Has this every happened before?

Finally let us look at the government actions. Before the vaccine people decried the shutdown of the economy. There was no treatment and no vaccine, so this was an alternative. As I mentioned before, I can understand protecting the old or compromised. These were at higher risk of dying. If we were not going to get a vaccine, it would be logical that to induce herd immunity, we would allow the healthy people who were low risk to be exposed to the virus to develop enough herd immunity, that is assuming those who were infected were protected from further infections, that it would eventually stop the epidemic and protect the older folks. Shutting down the economy did not do this and the damage which has occurred from this action is still developing.

If we had no vaccine, allowing children to go to school when it became evident that they were at low risk getting severe disease, would induce both innate and adaptive immunity to protect them in the future, and hasten the development of herd immunity,

Our government and CDC chose not to go this route and placed all out trust in a future vaccine. Of course, that entailed spending a lot of money and bypassing the normal route of FDA approval to get the vaccine out, but political pressure prevailed.

Once the vaccine was approved, we went all in and advised everyone to get the vaccine. We do that all the time with the flu vaccine, so no big deal. Just to make sure everyone was in the same boat; the vaccines were essentially mandated. You could not force people to get it, but you could not allow them to work, go to school, take transportation, or stay in the military. This was really just forcing them to take it.

I have a good memory of those times, after all it was only about two years ago. I do not recall any debate on the subject. Just the opposite. Any dissenting opinions were not allowed. Physicians echoed the government's position, although I know there were those who disagreed. The medical boards threatened physicians who objected. Most physicians are now involved in a group practice and the managers of these various practices did not allow dissent. The government-controlled social media did not allow any alternative positions. You could be fired for objecting to the vaccine.

As a result, it will end up that over 85% of the adults got vaccinated. With the current drive to vaccinate children, I anticipate a high percentage of them will end up vaccinated.

Dr. Bossche is quite adamant that this is a terrible idea and backs up his statements with scientific reasoning. The CDC has many cleaver scientists, some of these probably agree with him. You will not hear from any of them.

Over the last year there has been more information available. The government and social media sites have allowed information to flow. I believe in the common sense of most people if they are given information. Parents are particularly interested in their children. Over the last year they have been voting with their feet and the rate of children being vaccinated has dropped markedly. They simply do not trust the government, the CDC, physicians, or pediatric societies. None of these organizations will admit that perhaps they were wrong. This just extends the mistrust.

I don't know that if there was no vaccine and we allowed herd immunity to develop from natural infection, if the variants would have developed as rapidly. I think it is likely the vaccines hastened the development. If catching covid would prevent you from getting it again, herd immunity will have already occurred.

We are no closer to herd immunity. The government is spinning the data by saying we are now going to say herd immunity has occurred when the death rate is low. The same way they are spinning the definition of a successful vaccine.

Next month a new approved booster will be released. Already the variant that the booster is targeting is falling in incidence and now only accounts for about 25% of the cases. In a couple months it may be gone. Never the less, you will still see ads recommending you get it to keep from getting severe disease when they do not know why it would work, and probably the booster will have little protection.

Now let's move on to **WHAT IS GOING TO HAPPEN**.

WHAT IS GOING TO HAPPEN

The future is easy to predict but difficult to be accurate. This is a book about Dr. Bossche's paper. Unlike me, he is a real expert. He backs up his predictions with logic, biochemistry, and experience. Upon reading the paper you realize these are not general predictions but are very specific about the genotype evolutionary changes that are likely to occur. I have taught you the basics you need to understand to make rational decisions on the health of yourself and your family,

We all understand that mutations in the genome result in changing amino acids, deleting amino acids, or adding amino acids to the spike protein This virus seems to be partial to mutations and they are occurring all the time. Previously the Omicron virus developed increased infectivity secondary to the neutralizing antibodies not binding to the changed amino acids epitopes on the receptor binding domain. In addition, the virulence is decreased secondary to the non-neutralizing antibodies attached to portions of the N-terminal domain. If you have a mutation that changes this attachment, you will decrease infectiousness which will not be driving evolutionary dynamics.

The current prominent variants are offspring from Omicron.

Dr. Bossche asks the question " Could the virulence increase without decreasing the infectiousness?". In other words, could the virus become more deadly and just as infective if not more.

To answer this question, we must consider glycosylation.

N-linked glycosylation, the attachment of a carbohydrate consisting of several sugar molecules (glycan) to a nitrogen atom, which in our case is the amide nitrogen of the amino acid asparagine, found in the spike protein.

O-linked glycosylation is the attachment of a carbohydrate (glycan) to the oxygen atom of the amino acids, serine, or threonine. This is the more common one in the spike protein.

We have already gone over this process.

Like glycation (the attachment of a single sugar molecule to a protein or fat, glycosylation can be affected by the amount of glucose in the serum. That is those with type 2 diabetes, prediabetes, or obesity are likely to have higher glucose levels and hence more glycosylation. This may be a factor in the increased severity of disease in patients with these conditions.

Since Dr. Bossche and others believe the mass vaccination campaign has suppressed innate immunity, diminished interferon release, short-circuited any "training" of the immune system, and increased the infectiveness of the virus, he has a dismal outlook.

He believes.

A variant will develop which will be more infectious than Omicron yet have a high death rate.

Those vaccinated will not develop new IgG antibodies against this new virus.

As it is now, getting the new virus will not prevent re-infection.

The current vaccines will be quite ineffective against the new virus

The only way to stop the pandemic is through herd immunity. The only ones who can develop immunity are those who were not vaccinated and had a natural infection. These will be the ones who can train their innate immune system to be sensitized to these antigens and recall the trained cells after future exposure to these antigens.

Let me remind you that although the innate system does not develop specific antibodies, it does develop IgM antibodies which, although not specific to a particular antigen, can be trained to mount a vigorous response to these. Groups of antigens. In addition, the cytotoxic cells (NK) can be sensitized to these general antigens.

Recall antibodies are not antibiotics. They do not kill anything. An antibiotic can kill bacteria without killing the cell. An antibody marks the virion or infected cell so that the innate system can dispose of them.

The covid mRNA vaccine caused high levels of IgG to be developed before the innate system could become sensitized and thus educated. These recurrent high levels through repeat infections or vaccinations continue to suppress the innate system. The elevated IgG response to the antigen prevents any new variant IgG from being produced. Once you are covid vaccinated, you cannot become unvaccinated.

He believes the worst possible course is to vaccinate children, especially young children. Elevated IgG levels will prevent future development of the innate system, not only for covid but also impair any innate system education for other viruses. You cannot become covid unvaccinated.

He wants to:

Stop covid vaccinations.

Use chemical prophylaxis to prevent infection (none currently available)

Await the development of natural immunity in the population to get to the point of herd immunity. (Of course, what other option do we have)

The main controversy over Dr. Bossche's paper, and what the media seems to emphasize, are the predictions as to what will happen should this occur.

He concludes that the pandemic will only be resolved by herd immunity. This requires a strong innate immune system. The relevant IgMs are likely compromised in those who have been vaccinated. The adaptive system has failed in those individuals to provide sterilizing immunity.

This means the pandemic will continue to exist in highly vaccinated regions as long as we continue to boost non-neutralizing antibodies. One way to stop the pandemic would be effective anti-viral medicine that could be administered to the entire population; that is stop mass vaccination and start mass administration. Currently we have no such drug nor the capability to supply most of the population with one.

Herd immunity could occur naturally if:

1. A baby boom to start over with non-vaccinated individuals.
2. Mass immigration from poorly vaccinated countries
3. Evolution of the virus to a variant to one which would cause a high rate of severe disease and death in those who have immune suppression, that is those who have been vaccinated. When enough of these people have died, and the number of healthy, unvaccinated individuals can get high enough, then normal herd immunity will occur. That is, when the percentage of unvaccinated is higher than the percentage of vaccinated.

Many critics claim he is predicting Armageddon This is an event which occurs at the end of the tribulation, a time that does see many deaths from disease. The tribulation is followed by the 1000-year millennial kingdom, which ends in the destruction of a great army.

KELLY GREGG MD

WRAP UP

Now I will tell you what I think. Remember I am a retired physician and do not have a license to practice medicine, hence, anything I tell you is not medical advice. I will tell you what I advise my family or fellow church members to do, but I am not an expert.

Dr. Bossche did accomplish what I wished. That is, he provided a reasonable explanation as to why the covid deaths/cases graph looks the way it does. He did give a good explanation why herd immunity is not around the corner, no matter how many covid vaccines you get. I have given you enough information that now you can understand.

I believe most everyone involved in the science in this area will accept his logic and observations, at least in the first half of the paper. When you start predicting what is going to happen, you may get other opinions.

I do think the variants will continue to develop. It is quite possible a more virulent one will occur. It would not be reasonable to expect a less infectious variant of Omicron can surpass the current disease without some type of advantage.

I think we made a mistake in mandating the current covid vaccines. We were told everyone had to get it to prevent the spread of the virus. This did not turn out as advertised, and perhaps just the opposite. The more information that comes out reveals that all the side effects were not made known. They did not tell us the mRNA in the vaccine had undergone genetic modification. They did not tell us about the effects on the innate immune system, or the differences between the responses of this vaccine verses a natural infection, although this was probably known.

We know the reason why they did not tell us. If we had all the facts, many may have chosen not to get the vaccine. Hence there was a full court press to do whatever it took to get people vaccinated, even if we had to hide the truth a little bit. That turned out to not be enough and the vaccine became essentially mandated. This was done through fear, the way the government always tries to get its way when logical convincing is not enough.

I, like many people, got the vaccine. I cannot become unvaccinated. Now I must ride out the storm.

I do agree that covid vaccination of children is a terrible idea. There may be a few exceptions, but a very few. We forced everyone in the military to get vaccinated, probably the healthiest collection of people. We forced kids to get vaccinated to go to college. Some were forced to get vaccinated to go to school. It would not be surprising if we forced anyone attending kindergarten to get vaccinated, despite what we know about its effectiveness and risks.

I do not have as pessimistic an outlook as Dr. Bossche. There are many new vaccines in development and probably that many medications to treat or prevent covid. All we need is one that will keep you from getting infected or infecting anyone else and there is a chance for herd immunity. I agree this is the only way to get out of a pandemic.

Dr. Bossche also did mention a possible antigenic shift in the virus. Currently the variants are close enough to the original that getting a variant does not stimulate the adaptive system to make a brand-new different antibody.

Of course, if this happened, the vaccines would then become worthless, and the government would start mass vaccinations with a new vaccine all over again, and thus we would end up in the same place. That is unless this were a real vaccine that would work.

I am somewhat surprised that Dr. Bossche did not mention the possibility (from my point of view the probability) that covid is an intentionally genetically modified virus that was not derived from nature. This may explain why the vaccine did not work, or that even with an antigenic shift a vaccine would not work.

There continues to be suppression of alternative opinions and explanations. This is one reason I wrote this book.

What will I advise if what Dr. Bossche predicts begins to happen?

Let's start with our present state. If you are in a high-risk group, which means your immune system is diminished or you are older than 65, you may consider getting the boosters. As I mentioned, this will elevate the neutralizing antibodies and, even if they do not work well, will still provide some protection for a couple months.

Of course, you elevated the non-neutralizing antibodies which enhance your risk of getting infected, so there is a sweet spot when the higher antibodies balance the increased risk. This does not last long. Even if you get covid, the virulence of this variant is so low that the risk is small, especially for those who are young and normal.

If you get the vaccine, there may be a recommendation that you continue getting them every three months. There may come a time when even this does not protect those at high risk.

If you read carefully, you recognize that there may be other risks of taking the mRNA vaccine itself. It does appear that it diminishes the innate system and thus may predispose you to some other viral infection that might kill you. It also may adversely affect the role of cancer prevention by the immune system.

I will not take any boosters, unless legally mandated.

Now if you are younger than 65 and in good health, I would not get the vaccine or boosters There may be rare exceptions, but in general do not get it.

If you are very young, I would not take it for reasons explained by the paper.

Getting Omicron and having little risk is not because the neutralizing antibodies are working. It is because the non-neutralizing antibodies which increase infectiousness also reduces the chance of systemic spread. If the virion is attached to a dendritic cell, steric changes are produced in which the non-neutralizing antibodies to the NTD results in closure of the petal and thus decreased infectiveness as opposed to the effect on free virions which results in open petals and increased infectiveness.

If the next variant, which will be more infectious, results in a higher rate of severe disease, I may have to change my advice. If the next variant is completely resistant to the vaccine, then I will not advise anyone to get it. It would increase the risk of infection and not provide benefit.

The risk /benefit from taking the vaccine is difficult to determine in some individuals and is quite subjective and thus requires both knowledge of the patient's medical condition and evaluation of the current state of the vaccine. For young healthy patients it is easy, but as you get into higher risk group, it is more difficult and dynamic as the risk of the vaccine increases and the benefits decline.

It may be of greater benefit to increase the functioning of your innate system and do what you can to enhance your body's normal reparative processes. If what Dr. Bossche predicts comes to pass, this will be the only treatment.

My main interest is Diet and Health. If you want to do something to decrease your risk of death and you are in a higher risk category, get your obesity, prediabetes, and type 2 diabetes under control. I have detailed how to do this at length in other books.

Then consider the benefits of fasting. It is something everyone can do. Stop eating after dinner one day, do not eat anything the next day, and eat breakfast the following day. Do this two non-consecutive days a week. See Fasting and Autophagy for the Common Man.

I usually do not advise extra vitamins and supplements. As long as we are in the pandemic, I advise anyone over age 55 or who is immune compromised to take 5000 units of vitamin D a day. I do not really like to recommend this, but I have become convinced this will help your innate immune system and possibly prevent death if you get covid. I am not sure if it will prevent getting covid, but it probably will markedly lessen your risk of dying if you do.

If you are not in the high-risk category, take vitamin D if you have been tested and your level is less than 50 ng/ml., or if you get covid.

I changed my mind. Take vitamin D 5000 units a day in the summer, and 10,000 units a day in the fall and winter. This medication is cheap and has very few side effects. Do not take more than 10,00o units a day. More is not better.

If you have a two-year-old, consider a BCG vaccine. No one in the US knows much about BCG, although it is commonly used in the rest of the world. There is increasing evidence this will help with covid and I predict it will start being offered in some pediatric practices. Become more educated before you give your child the vaccine.

Make sure you talk to your pediatrician about this. The BCG vaccine does convert your PPD to positive. I think it may be more important to just not give your normal child a covid vaccine. Let your child be normal and do not have them wear a mask.

There are other things you can do to prevent covid or treat an early case of covid.

I advise you to look up FLCCC, Front Line Covid-19 Critical Care Alliance

This will provide protocols for prevention and early treatment of covid, and probably will be of benefit if the new, deadlier covid appears.

https://covid19criticalcare.com/covid-19-protocols/

Above all, use your common sense. You now know a lot more about covid than when you started.

Things change and new information will be generated. Dr. Bossche may not be entirely correct about the future, but I think his explanation about what is happening right now is correct.

The information in this field is rapidly changing I will edit this book every couple months as the paperback books are printed on demand. This enables me to easily update the content.

Ivermectin has been used early in a covid infection to possibly ameliorate the infection. Recent studies do not show a significant advantage to using the drug. However, there continues to be confusion with the studies as it is uncertain if the correct dose was used. It is difficult to explain away the positive results from millions of people taking this drug in India. Right now, I would take the middle road, that is, if you are at high risk and get covid, take the drug. If you are low risk, think about it. If covid is killing a bunch of people, take it, if you can find it.

Hydroxychloroquine may be of some use. This drug enhances the absorption of zinc in the cell so take zinc with it.

Lipitor (atorvastatin) has shown beneficial effects It is a safe, cheap drug with minimal side effects Although these are early findings, if you are at high risk for getting covid, you may want to consider taking the drug (40 mg daily) or if you contact covid you may want to take it a couple weeks. Many people are already on this drug. If the death rate goes up, take the drug.

As time has gone on, I am not sure how much of an advantage you will get taking Lipitor. If you are on it, do not stop. If the mortality rate of covid rises, people are going to be doing all kinds of things like taking mega-doses of vitamins. I would rather try Lipitor, especially as there will be a huge demand for vitamins.

The covid vaccine induced the production of many spike protein antigens, more than a natural infection. You have a high level of these antigens, and a high level of these antibodies, The spike protein has been found in exosomes. Exosomes are 200 nm size vesicles generated by cells which serve as a method by which cells in your body communicate.

We know that the spike protein is contained in exosomes and can stimulate antibody attachment. The vaccine has stimulated a large number of antigens (from the spike protein) which means a more vigorous and prolonged stimulation of the immune system resulting in a constant inflammatory state. We may be seeing the results of this state over the next year. I mention this as it may impact your decision to get the booster. We are always considering the risk/benefit of the vaccine. This goes on the risk side of the equation.

There have now been numerous reports of excess deaths. That is deaths above the normal incidence even after you remove the covid deaths. These are in the range of a 10%-20% increase. It does appear that these excess deaths are more common in those countries that have a high vaccination rate. We have suspected the mass vaccination of mRNA vaccines may depress your innate system somewhat such that you may have an increased risk of cancer or other diseases.

It does appear taking Paxlovid may be useful in preventing severe disease. You take this within five days of the diagnosis and take the medication for five days. Studies are being done on the current variants which still have a low risk of severity.

If a new more virulent variant arises, I am not sure how much Paxlovid will help. It may not make a difference as taking Paxlovid will be one of the things people will try if the mortality increases and there will be a huge demand and you probably will not be able to get it.

Of course if the mortality increases, all kinds of things will be tried as we really do not have a good treatment for the disease. We end up back to supportive therapy.

I'm sure I will be able to buy snake oil somewhere.

Paxlovid is free if you have a positive covid test. If you do not, it costs about $500 for a cycle. Paxlovid is not approved for preventive therapy, but that will not stop people from taking it daily for months.

I have decided not to write a chapter on long covid. At this point there is simply not enough information I trust that I can teach you anything that would be of value to you.

I am not a licensed physicians and this is not medical advice. These are my opinions based upon my life time accumulation of knowledge and common sense. Although this is not medical advice, once you read the book, you will know more about the subject and may consider this to be good advice.

Although it has not occurred, I still am in agreement with Dr. Bossche that it is inevitable that a more virulent, more infective variant will arrive.

It appears that about 80% of the people in the USA have been vaccinated, and about 100% show evidence of having had a previous covid infection. The variants continue to be quite infectious, whether you have had a vaccine or not. The mortality is around.1%, whether you have had a vaccine or not. As always, the mortality is higher in older, high risk, obese patients.

Almost everyone I know has had a vaccine and/or had covid, so I really hope Dr. Bossche's prediction does not happen. Never the less, I believe it will unless some dramatic medical treatment arrives.

I have been vaccinated and I cannot become unvaccinated. Those who are not vaccinated will have a greater chance to survive. Right now I advise almost no one to get a vaccine. Right now I advise almost no children to get a vaccine.

Remember I am not a licensed physician, so my medical advice means nothing.

As I mentioned, I have an interest in diet and health. We know obesity, which often is present in those with Type 2 diabetes, is a marked risk factor of death from covid. I have written much on how to prevent or treat obesity in an effort to reduce the incidence of T2DM.

Many of the complications of covid seem to be related to activation of the immune system, perhaps through induction of inflammation via the spike protein As I have said, I and many others have been vaccinated, and hence subject to the increased risks of both catching covid and dying of covid secondary to the depression of my innate system.

Vitamin D may be somewhat effective in enhancing or at least boosting the immune system.

Paxlovid may or may not be useful in preventing severe disease, but I do not know if it will work well at all if there is a new, more virulent variant.

How can I assist those who may catch a new variant, or really help them that get covid at all.

It does appear elevated leptin and interleukin-6 does play a role in severity of the disease. We already know obesity and T2DM is a factor. If you get covid, it is not reasonable to tell you to lose fat or get rid of T2DM. All of these people have already tried to do that but failed. You are not going to lose much fat in the couple weeks after getting covid.

I am a fasting advocate. I have written Fasting and Autophagy for the Common Man. I do know that the leptin levels drop markedly withing a couple days of fasting. I do think that elevated leptin levels seem to induce the production of Interleukin-6 which seems to be closely related to the complications of covid infections. It has been suggested that lowering the leptin may improve the prognosis.

What I am saying is why not advise those higher risk patients, and perhaps all patients, to begin fasting when they get the diagnosis. Not eating for a week will not harm you. It will lower your leptin level.

If we do get a more virulent variant, it is unlikely there will be any good treatment. How about just stopping eating?

Paperback Books
Diet and Health
Diabetes, Prediabetes Obesity
Ketogenic Diet for Beginners
Fasting and Autophagy
Maintenance Diet
Bread In the Modern Diet
Epigenetics In Pregnancy
Introduction to Cell Biology and Epigenetics
Diet and Disaster: Food Shortage
Covid and Vaccines for Medical Professionals
Covid and Vaccines for the Common Man
Allulose and Other Sweeteners
Practical Sex for Older Married Couples
Sexuality in Marriage After Fifty
eBook A2 Milk
eBook Brain Disease and Fasting
eBook Tampons and Cancer
eBook Let's Rename PCOS
eBook Weight Loss for Women
eBook-Fat Kids and Fasting
eBook Lipoproteins in Diet and Health
eBook Autophagy and Ages
eBook Carbs for Food Engineers
eBook Fructose and Soy for Food Engineers
eBook Fasting and Disease
eBook Know Your Orgasm
(for advertising Know Your Organ)
eBook Know Your Masturbation
(for advertising Find Yourself)
eBook Know Your Clitoris
(for advertising Know Yourself)

eBook Artificial Sweeteners and the Gut Biome
eBook 28 Day Fast
eBook Dementia in Women
eBook Fat and Protein for Food Engineers
eBook The Food Engineer
eBook Flour Treatment
eBook Bread Gluten and Sensitivity
eBook Introduction to Stem Cell
(Regenerative Cell) Treatment
eBook Prolonged Fasting